Praise for *The Compassionate Mind Approach to Building Self-Confidence:*

'This book will help you stop undermining yourself with debilitating self-criticism and start giving yourself the same kindness, encouragement and support you'd give to a good friend. With straightforward explanations of concepts and dozens of easy and practical exercises to "build self-confidence" through self-compassion, this book has the power to change your life.'

Kristin Neff, PhD, author of *Self-Compassion*; Associate Professor, University of Texas at Austin

'Compassionate Mind approaches are one of the most exciting developments in cognitive behaviour therapy. Mary Welford has written an easy to read, interactive book that distils the core features of developing a different relationship with one's mind and paradoxically building one's self-confidence.'

Professor David Veale, Institute of Psychiatry, King's College London

'Hugely approachable, sympathetic and fun. I'd recommend this book to anyone wanting to improve their self-confidence. Chock-full of brilliant clinical metaphors and creative techniques, it will also be invaluable to any therapist wanting a primer on this fascinating area.'

Dr Sam Cartwright-Hatton, Clinical Psychologist and NIHR Fellow, University of Sussex

'This is a wonderful book! Dr Welford has beautifully written a remarkable book that takes us to the heart of building self-confidence through developing self-compassion. This book is based on a robust science of mind that leads directly to sensitive and kind-hearted understanding of how we develop self-critical ways of coping with difficult and stressful life experiences. This book enables you to develop an empathic understanding of the origins of shame and also provides practical skills and techniques in developing a compassionate mind as the basis for self-confidence. This book is a highly accessible and practically useful means of developing and overcoming obstacles to self-compassion.'

Professor Andrew Gumley, University of Glasgow, UK

'Dr Mary Welford's book is helpful, informative and interesting. The book makes you feel very much "looked after", and the inclusion of personal stories, including her own, gives the reader a sense of not being on their own. The approach is hugely relevant to those wishing to find their compassionate self and build their self-confidence.'

Erica Wakeman, reader

THE COMPASSIONATE MIND APPROACH TO BUILDING SELF-CONFIDENCE

MARY WELFORD

ROBINSON

ROBINSON

First published in Great Britain by Robinson in 2012

9 10

Important Note
This book is not intended as a substitute for medical advice or
treatment. Any person with a condition requiring medical attention
should consult a qualified medical practitioner or suitable therapist.

A CIP catalogue record for this book
is available from the British Library.

ISBN: 978-1-78033-032-7

Printed in Italy by Elcograf S.p.A.

Papers used by Robinson are from well-managed forests
and other responsible sources

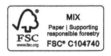

Robinson
An imprint of
Little, Brown Book Group
Carmelite House
50 Victoria Embankment
London EC4Y 0DZ

The authorised representative
in the EEA is
Hachette Ireland
8 Castlecourt Centre
Dublin 15, D15 XTP3, Ireland
(email: info@hbgi.ie)

An Hachette UK Company
www.hachette.co.uk

www.littlebrown.co.uk

Contents

Foreword

We have always understood that compassion is very important. The way we feel about ourselves and the way we think other people feel about us has a huge impact on our well-being. If we value and support ourselves we are more likely to successfully negotiate all that life throws at us. This is in contrast to being self-critical and feeling that there's something wrong with us. However, it is not just common sense that tells us about the value of compassion. Recent advances in scientific studies have greatly developed our understanding of how compassion, both from ourselves and from others, can help us to treat ourselves in ways that are respectful and improve our sense of well-being.

We live in a world where we are constantly advised to judge, rate and evaluate ourselves. All around us are messages that we might not be good enough. Maybe our parents told us such things or maybe at school we were often the last one to be picked for the team. Of course, nowadays schools are constantly focused on tests, judgements and evaluations of all kinds. Over the last ten to twenty years, even competitions on television have become increasingly focused on which contestant will be thrown off the show. From *Big Brother* to cookery competitions, we see people anxiously waiting to find out if they will be the one voted off, the camera following those recently ejected in their tearful departures. This may well be good for television, but it doesn't do a lot for our psychological well-being. It fosters the old view that only success and achieving and doing things can make us happy, and if we are not up to scratch or we do something wrong then we too will feel anxious, unhappy and tearful. So it doesn't take much to recognize that our sense of belonging and community can be a lot more fragile than it used to be. Indeed our focus on self-esteem and achievement, at the expense of helping, sharing and nurturing our community, has been offered as one reason why depression and anxiety are on the increase in the modern world, especially amongst younger people.

What research tells us, however, is that if we learn to value and respect ourselves, if we treat ourselves and others with kindness even when things are going wrong, we are much more likely to be able to cope with setbacks and to be happier. Whilst striving for success is important, seeking to be compassionate to yourself and to others has been shown time and again to be associated with a sense of well-being. After all, it's easy to become critical, harsh and rejecting when things go wrong, but the real measure of ourselves is whether we can be supportive and encouraging when life is tough.

In this important book, Dr Mary Welford uses her wealth of experience and knowledge in working with people with a whole range of psychological difficulties. She explores why our brains are so susceptible to reacting to life setbacks and difficulties in the way that they do and especially why we have a tendency to judge ourselves and be self-critical. Unlike other animals, we have a brain that is constantly thinking and judging. Imagine the zebra running away from a lion. Once the zebra has escaped, it will shortly settle down to feed again. However, this may not happen in humans because we can spend many days ruminating about what would have happened if we had got caught and fantasizing about the most horrible things. Zebras and chimpanzees don't worry about what they're thinking, what they look like or what other chimpanzees might be thinking about them! Humans, on the other hand, do – and all the time! We look in the mirror and think, 'Oh gosh, is that really me? How come I have put on so much weight?' Of course, we also think about our internal worlds – the fantasies, thoughts and feelings we have within us – and we can be critical of those too. Life becomes full of shoulds and shouldn'ts or oughts and ought nots or even musts and must nots. Again, no other animal thinks, judges, dislikes, fears or tries to avoid their fantasies, feelings and thoughts in the way that humans do. We call this self-criticism, and many people who struggle with self-confidence can be harsh and self-critical towards themselves. By slowing down it is possible to really explore the nature of our self-criticism and realize how constant and unpleasant it can be.

Now, of course, there are times when we certainly want to be aware of our mistakes and to improve. It's not that we are never disappointed with how things turn out, but it's more how we deal with this disappointment. Do we deal with it openly, honestly, kindly and supportively or harshly and aggressively, which actually makes us feel much worse? Compassion, as we will see, is not about being slapdash and careless; rather, it is about being generally supportive and encouraging to do our best!

Dr Welford helps us to understand that our susceptibility to getting caught up in negative ways of feeling and thinking about ourselves can be very unhelpful. She also helps us to recognize that, because of the way our brains are designed, it's relatively easy for us to get into the habit of putting ourselves down. Indeed, this is a universal human trait and abso-lutely *not our fault*. After all, we didn't design our brains with their various capacities for emotions, thoughts and fantasies. Nor did we design our capacities for complex thinking, and ruminating. And nor did we choose our backgrounds or our genes, both of which can make us more or less susceptible to being kind and supportive or critical of ourselves.

We all have different genes, talents, and abilities, and we come from a whole range of backgrounds. All these serve to make us slightly different from each other. So while some people are highly intelligent and win Nobel prizes, others are less so and struggle with basic reading and writ-ing; while some people are great conversationalists, others are shy and struggle with what to say. A key message in this book, therefore, is that we all simply find ourselves 'here' and, whatever 'the slings and arrows of outrageous fortune', our relationship with ourselves is very important for how we cope with life. Research shows that the more compassion-ate we are towards ourselves, the happier we are, and the more resilient we become when faced with difficulties in our lives. In addition, we are better able to reach out to others for help, and feel more compassionate towards other people too, making us good to have as a friend.

Compassion can sometimes be viewed as being a bit 'soft' or 'weak', a question of just 'being nice' or 'letting your guard down' and 'not trying hard enough'. *This is a major mistake* because, on the contrary, compassion requires us to be courageous and sometimes to be open to our painful feelings and to learn to tolerate them, to face up to our own problematic emotions and difficulties and the disappointments we can have of ourselves. Compassion does not mean turning away from emotional difficulties or discomforts, or trying to get rid of them. Compassion means noticing when we have been critical of ourselves and acted in potentially unhelpful ways and then making a deliberate choice to be compassionate, generating inner support and encouragement. So, it is *not* a soft option; rather, compassion simply means being sensitive and aware of our distress (and of the distress of others) with a genuine commitment to try to do something about it. There is nothing soft or weak in either of those two efforts. So, in fact, compassion helps us to build courage, honesty and commitment to learn to cope with the difficulties we face. It enables us to do things to and for ourselves that help us to flourish and take care of ourselves – not as a demand or requirement, but to enable us to live our lives more fully and contentedly.

In this book Dr Welford draws on her many years of experience as a clinical psychologist and psychotherapist, working with people who often feel bad about themselves for one reason or another. Maybe they carry shame from the past or are just disappointed that they can't be the way they wish to be or more in control of their emotions. Dr Welford outlines a model of compassion that seeks to stimulate and build our self-confidence so that we can engage with things that we find difficult. She helps us learn how to develop a supportive friendship with ourselves that will help us when times are difficult.

The approach that Dr Welford takes is called a Compassionate *Mind* Approach because when we engage compassion it can influence our attention, thoughts, feelings and behaviour; in other words, how our mind operates *as a whole*. The Compassionate Mind Approach draws on many other well-developed approaches, including those of Eastern traditions such as Buddhism. In addition, Compassionate Mind Approaches, especially those that form part of Compassion Focused Therapy as seen here, are rooted in scientific understanding of how our mind works.

Undoubtedly, over the years our understanding of compassion and how to promote it will change and improve. One thing that doesn't change, however, is the fact that kindness, warmth and understanding go a long way towards helping us when we suffer. In these pages you will find these qualities in abundance so you too can learn to be gentle, understanding, supportive and kind but also engaging and courageous when working through difficulties.

Many people suffer silently and secretly with a whole range of problems that can be linked to a lack of self-confidence and a tendency to be self-critical. Some feel ashamed or angry with themselves, others sometimes feel fearful of not being able to cope in particular ways. Sadly, shame can stop many of us from reaching out for help. But, by opening your heart to compassion, and recognizing our common humanity and vulnerability to suffering, we can take the first steps towards dealing with these difficulties in new and more effective ways. My compassionate wishes go with you on your journey.

Professor Paul Gilbert PhD FBPsS OBE

March 2012

Author's Note

In years gone by I would have been unable to hand over the final draft of a book without experiencing crippling self-criticism. Today I can hold my self-criticism at bay and acknowledge the fact that this book is by no means perfect, but *it is the best I can do at this moment in time and that's OK*. The application of this approach to my personal life has taught me this, for which I am truly thankful. This is just one of the reasons why I sincerely recommend it to others.

Preface

Compassion Focused Therapy (CFT) was developed by Professor Paul Gilbert of Derbyshire, UK. The 'compassionate mind approach' has been developed to describe aspects of this therapy that may be used as 'self-help'. Paul has both helped and worked alongside a large number of people experiencing difficulties. He has also taught, supervised and mentored a team of therapists and researchers, who have been able to contribute to the development of the therapy. I am privileged to say I am part of this team.

The compassionate mind approach is informed by a wide range of theories and areas of research, such as evolution, neuroscience and psychology. It also uses a range of exercises that have been found to be helpful. Although some have been drawn from Eastern traditions, such as Buddhism, it is important to note that in CFT such exercises have been isolated from their religious or spiritual origins and are used on a purely secular basis.

In the compassionate mind approach we aim to build self-confidence through the development of self-compassion and choose not to focus on concepts such as 'self-esteem'. (It's not that we think the term self-esteem is necessarily unhelpful, but we tend to view it more as the natural outcome of having *built* self-confidence.)

There are many definitions of self-esteem but these are often linked to the feeling that you have achieved certain life goals and that, compared with other people, you're doing OK. Work on self-esteem can therefore involve improving how you feel *in comparison* with others. When things are going well we can feel good about ourselves, but when we fall short of our own expectations, or those of others, we are prone to feeling bad. Although an improvement in self-esteem may be what you feel you want right now, in this book we are going to focus on self-compassion as a major tool towards building your self-confidence. In contrast to self-esteem, self-confidence and self-compassion come to the fore when things are going badly.[1]

Evolution: fact or fiction?

We all have different beliefs and it is understandable that not everyone reading this will believe the same things as I do. I obviously want to respect different views but also be true to how I see things. I believe in evolution. I personally believe that we have evolved from single-celled organisms, from reptiles and from apes. I believe that 'natural selection' had a central role in driving evolution, making certain traits, characteristics, physical attributes and skills more common and others less so. However, I am also aware that natural selection may not be the only influencing factor in this process. It might not be the only thing that accounts for how we are today. I personally believe that other answers will come from science but I am also aware that we may not know 'for sure'.

Some people believe that something or someone else had a role to play in the process of evolution and has guided things. Others believe that human beings were created and are not descended from any other animal life. If these or any other beliefs make you question what is written here, please do not simply turn away.

Hopefully, we can agree that we all have a very complicated brain that has evolved at least since human beings existed (and that in itself is a very long time). In addition, our brain development is influenced by our experiences, and we will look at this in a lot more detail later. As such, our brain is equipped with many amazing capacities but with many difficult and conflicting things as well, all of which we have to deal with and work out. I hope that agreeing this may assist those who don't believe in evolution to still get something out of this book.

---

[1]   If you're interested you can look at Kristin Neff's website (www.self-compassion. org) for further discussion of the distinction between self-compassion and self-esteem.

Self-compassion, in particular, helps us think about ourselves as being similar to other people with the same difficulties, rather than judging ourselves against them. Self-compassion both encourages us and provides us with a way of supporting ourselves. It doesn't depend on being successful, in the way that self-esteem might, or on being overly optimistic. Self-compassion helps us to treat ourselves in a way that brings out our best qualities. As we will see, it's no easy option – it can be quite tough, in fact – but the aim of this book is to help *build self-confidence through self-compassion*.

It starts by outlining the way in which the compassionate mind approach views self-confidence. With a better understanding of how the human emotional systems behave and regulate each other, you will be made aware of how you may be undermining yourself. To counteract this you will then be guided through a range of exercises aimed at building your self-confidence.

How to Use This Book

When is it best to do this work?

'The time to repair the roof is when the sun is shining'

– J. F. Kennedy, 87th State of the Union Address, 1962

If you decided to learn to swim it wouldn't be advisable to throw yourself in at the deep end. Instead you would probably start by going to your local pool at a quiet time, getting into the shallow end, and gradually progressing to more and more difficult challenges as you built up your confidence with being in the water.

It may be helpful for you to think about how you go about following the exercises in this book in a similar way. In other words, start gradually, when things are relatively 'easy' for you. I use this term very loosely because, of course, life is very rarely easy, but it is likely that there are some times in your day, week, month or even year that are better suited to certain tasks than others. Choose to start when you can predict things will be less hectic and you will have the time and space to focus your efforts.

Take your time

One of the fundamental principles guiding the compassionate mind approach is that *intellectual* understanding does not necessarily bring about *emotional* change. In other words, while on an intellectual level we may *know* that we are loved or accepted by others, on an emotional level we may not *feel* it. Although many of the exercises in this book aim to address this gap between thinking and feeling, potentially one of the most powerful things you can do throughout this work is to take time to reflect and allow what you have learnt to 'sink in'. In other words, think about how the information you have been given relates to *you* and your own situation, regularly pausing to consider this for seconds, minutes, hours or longer.

Make a record of this process too. Something as simple as writing notes, and reviewing them in the future, can help you further narrow the gap between knowing something and feeling it.

Practical preparation

This book incorporates a number of worksheets, additional copies of which are freely available from the Compassionate Mind website (www. compassionatemind.co.uk). To supplement the worksheets I would encourage you to purchase, find or make a journal or notebook in which you can keep ongoing notes and reflections. In addition, you can use it for exercises such as writing compassionate letters.

Many people find it helpful always to use a specific pen or pencil when undertaking these tasks. I personally associate Biros with work and they can therefore trigger associated thoughts or feelings. For this reason I always use a fibre-tip pen when writing my journal. View these items as props to support you in building your self-confidence. In years to come they will act as a reminder of how far you have come in the development of your self-confidence and as a prompt for the practices it may be helpful for you to continue.

Book structure

The book consists of two key stages. The first involves looking at the concept of self-confidence in the context of our evolution, biology and life experiences. This will be the main focus of Chapters 1 to 3. The second stage involves exercises that help to build self-confidence by the application of self-compassion.

In the last chapter you will be encouraged to reflect upon which parts you have found most helpful, and utilize these to continue building your self-confidence in the future. In order to help you with this a personal practice summary sheet, containing a list of all the exercises that may be beneficial to you, is provided on pages xxviii–xxxii. Next to each exercise, space has been left for you to make notes on how useful you found it and any additional thoughts for your future guidance. Some of the exercises included here may be things you choose to do daily or weekly, while others may be things you do much less frequently.[2]

Finally, although self-help can be beneficial, in some circumstances it may not be enough. There is no shame in this – it's the reason why friends and family members confide in each other, and why I and thousands of other psychological therapists have jobs. At such times we can all best help ourselves by requesting or accepting help from others, be they friends, family or professionals. If you think you require professional help, speak to your General Practitioner who should be able to advise you about the options open to you.

---

[2] This book also contains a range of exercises that are not included in the summary sheet. This is because they are not to be used as 'personal practice', but instead illustrate and illuminate particular points raised by the author, to aid reflection on the reader's journey, or to help them work through initial obstacles.

Personal practice summary sheets

Exercise title	Usefulness	Additional notes
Mindfulness of sound		
Mindfulness of bodily sensations		
Mindfulness of breathing		
Mindfulness of a visual anchor point		
Mindfulness of a tactile anchor point		
Mindful walking		
Soothing rhythm breathing		
Finding your place of contentment		

Exercise title	Usefulness	Additional notes
Being deeply compassionate		
Re-experiencing your own compassion		
The ideal compassionate self		
Evoking a memory of compassion from others		
Turning compassion outwards		
Compassion for those who lack self-confidence		
Turning compassion inwards		
Compassion for your own journey and situation		

Exercise title	Usefulness	Additional notes
Developing your compassionate coach		
Recognizing thoughts and images that *have* occupied your mind		
Noticing thoughts and images *as* they occur in your mind		
Giving your new and compassionate brain a voice		
Two chairs		
Compassionate letter writing to build your self-confidence		
Compassionate letter writing *from* the compassionate role *to* yourself		
Writing a compassionate letter based on a compassionate alternative thoughts/images worksheet		
Identifying your own personal goals with respect to building your self-confidence		

Exercise title	Usefulness	Additional notes
Identifying the steps you need to take in working towards a goal		
Preparing to take action in social situations: using compassionate imagery I		
Preparing to take action: using compassionate imagery II		
Preparing to take action: using a compassionate alternative thoughts/images worksheet		
Preparing to take action: accessing inner support using compassionate letter writing		
Preparing to take action: compassionate behavioural experiment worksheets		
Doing your compassionate behavioural experiment		
Reviewing your compassionate behavioural experiment		
Communicating how we feel and what our needs are		

Exercise title	Usefulness	Additional notes
Giving constructive feedback		
Making seemingly small changes		
Savouring positive experiences		
Accepting yourself and things that you cannot change		
Embracing who you are		
Accepting your situation, right here, right now		
Guiding your day		
Using self-compassion in difficult situations		
Updating your formulation		
My personal plan for the future		

1 Self-confidence is Something We Build and Maintain, Not Something We Have

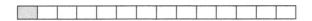

Our level of self-confidence can have a huge impact on the way things turn out for us. Take Jim, for example. He wanted to ask Becky out, but when he bumped into her his self-confidence failed him. Instead of suggesting they go out, he ended up talking about something completely different. 'What an idiot!' he told himself afterwards. Whether it be taking exams, going for job interviews, sorting out conflicts, taking up a new hobby, making friends, or any other form of initiative-taking, the outcome can be greatly influenced by the level of self-confidence with which we approach the task. And all of us, at some point in our lives, feel we could do with a bit more of it.

So what is self-confidence? If you look in a dictionary you'll find definitions such as 'trusting in one's abilities', 'having belief in oneself' or 'having assurance in oneself'. Self-confidence is actually difficult to define because it will differ from person to person. It may be summarised as the way each person *feels* about him or herself, in relation either to things they want to do or their own persona.

You will probably have noticed that your self-confidence varies from day to day, situation to situation. In certain arenas we can feel very self-confident, yet in others we feel almost exactly the opposite. Sometimes we find that in two seemingly similar situations our self-confidence levels vary widely. This can be both puzzling and frustrating.

But our self-confidence is not restricted to the way we react in certain situations, or how we believe we will be perceived by others. Self-confidence in relation to our own personality, thoughts and feelings, the things we like about ourselves and the things we don't, can greatly influence the lives we lead.

Where Does It All Start?

While it is true that some babies *seem* naturally more sociable and robust than others, it is difficult to pinpoint exactly where this starts. It is likely to be influenced by our genetics, time in the womb and experiences in the early days and weeks post-birth. However, for all of us, the interesting thing about self-confidence is that we all *build* it by first not having any. Think about how you first learnt to walk. It is likely that you initially struggled to your feet, fell over, cried, and then got to your feet once more. This will have happened over and over again until eventually you were running about and climbing trees.

In those early days you just *knew* what to do, and this helped build your self-confidence. What happens later on, in our adult lives? How would/ did you develop the self-confidence to drive a car, for instance? After all, almost everyone who finds themselves behind the wheel of a car for the first time will lack self-confidence, and anxiety may be 'sky high'.

But step by step, by continuing to learn despite your anxiety, self-confidence builds until eventually you become a reasonable driver. So building self-confidence is about developing ourselves by *doing* things despite our anxiety.

This is one of the key principles of this book – *self-confidence is something we build*. Even if you are starting from the point of having little or no self-confidence in a specific area, or indeed a range of different situations, with time and effort there is great potential for change. You *can* build your self-confidence.

However, like many things in life *self-confidence is something we also need to work to maintain*. And so this book is all about the processes by which we first build and then maintain self-confidence.

The First Secret of Building Self-confidence: Beware of Your Own Undermining

Before we look in more detail at the ways in which self-confidence is built, we need to be aware of a very important fact. One of the reasons we may lack self-confidence is because we ourselves actually undermine it – we simply don't allow it to grow and develop. Indeed one of the key things that we will explore in this book is how and why we *undermine* our own self-confidence, and what we can do to prevent this from happening.

Let's consider the case of Jim again. On the spot, and faced with Becky, he felt anxious and panicked by the situation. With images and thoughts about himself running through his mind, he imagined he looked awkward, red-faced, clammy and stupid. He thought to himself: 'There's no point in trying, I'll only make a hash of it. Who would want to go out with me anyway? She's bound to say no.' So rather than risk this outcome he avoided asking her.

In contrast, now imagine that in the days or weeks before bumping into Becky, whenever Jim pondered asking her out, he had thought to himself: 'This is going to be difficult, so I'll practise what to say . . . talk to a friend . . . get some advice.' If Jim had been able to do this, the outcome might have been very different.

Most people will be able to empathize with aspects of Jim's undermining thoughts but notice that when he is able to generate inner support he realizes and acknowledges both his anxiety and his lack of self-confidence. It is not that he is suddenly super-confident and free of anxiety. Instead he recognizes it is going to be difficult and works through, in a self-supportive way, how he can prepare and approach it. This is in marked contrast to the way he previously undermined his own self-confidence by telling himself rather unpleasant things.

As another example of self-undermining, imagine learning to drive while constantly telling yourself: 'I'll never get the hang of this . . . I'm bound to crash . . . the instructor's just not telling me how bad I am because she wants her weekly fee.' This way of thinking can't help but undermine you and make you feel much more anxious than you need to be. Of course it is not just our thoughts that can undermine us in such a situation; often it is how we *feel* about ourselves that can be our own undoing. If we feel stupid, inept and incompetent, this can, in turn, lead to undermining thoughts, images, and debilitating anxiety.

By contrast, suppose you think to yourself: 'It's perfectly normal to feel anxious, crash the gears, bump into the kerb and have cars blowing their horns at me – I am a learner after all.' Imagine simultaneously viewing that scenario with a sense of courage, acceptance and empathy for your own situation. If this were the case you would be far more likely to be able to ride the ups and downs of the learning process successfully.

The Second Secret of Building Self-confidence: Self-compassion

During the course of this book we are going to talk a lot about *self-compassion* so at this point it would be helpful to consider what does and does not constitute compassion.

People have a range of ideas about compassion. The simplest definition is a sensitivity to the pain (be it psychological or physical) that we and/or others may experience *plus* a motivation and genuine commitment to relieve it. It is the latter part of this definition that is most often overlooked. People often omit the more active component of compassion while emphasizing its elements such as kindness, warmth[3] and gentleness.[4]

While in certain situations self-compassion may predominantly involve these qualities, the compassionate mind approach also stresses the

---

[3] The term 'warmth' within the context of compassion refers to a sense of emotional warmth (rather than temperature!).
[4] It is also worth noting that many cultures define the word 'compassion' slightly differently. In Chapter 5 we will look at this in more detail.

importance of other key aspects of compassion – such as our ability to encourage, support and even push ourselves at the appropriate times. Self-compassion is not about sitting in a bath surrounded by candles, buying yourself some flowers, or treating yourself to something lovely to eat – or not unless such things are in your best interests. Self-compassion is about recognizing when we are struggling, and making a commitment to do what we can to improve things for ourselves, step by step. As such, it may involve making a commitment to get fit, eat a healthier diet or develop a hobby. It may involve facing a specific situation despite feeling high levels of anxiety, or letting yourself cry or feel angry about something that has happened because you need and deserve to do so. It may also be about addressing problems with drinking, drugs or overeating,[5] or anything else that is holding you back in life.

To illustrate this, let's think about Helen. She had been suffering from agoraphobia and had been a prisoner in her own house for over ten years without having the self-confidence to address the problem. Developing self-compassion did not involve her saying 'There there, never mind', and then surfing the net to buy herself lots of lovely things to compensate. Developing self-compassion in Helen's case meant warmly acknowledging that, in her own best interests, things needed to change. Self-compassion then involved her taking courageous steps to build her self-confidence in this respect, until eventually she opened her front door and stepped out on to the street despite feeling intense fear. Self-compassion for her meant that she reassured herself when things went wrong, recognized the difficult steps she was taking, and then courageously continued towards her goal.

---

[5]   If you want to know more about this, Kenneth Goss has written a book for the Compassionate Mind series specifically looking at ways of addressing overeating: *The Compassionate Mind Approach to Beating Overeating.*

Conclusions

In this opening chapter we have seen that self-confidence is something we build – not something we are simply born with. The way we go about building our self-confidence is crucial because we all need to be able to function while living with anxiety and uncertainty. It's this process of how we keep going when things get difficult for us that is central to the compassionate mind approach. By learning how to be compassionate to yourself, you will have a greater chance of building the self-confidence that will sustain you in times of difficulty.

And finally...

Having read this first chapter, and at the end of each subsequent one, I would encourage you to take some time to reflect on it and make a few notes in your journal or notebook. These may be on points you particularly wish to remember or on the way in which you think the topics discussed in this chapter may apply to you personally.

2 Understanding the Impact of Evolution on Us

The compassionate mind approach views all organisms on the planet as belonging to what Paul Gilbert terms 'the *flow of life*'. In other words, human beings are viewed as existing here in their current form by virtue of evolution – in just the same way as every other species on earth has evolved. If you look at the natural world around you, you will see animals competing for and fighting over status and territory, vying for food and for mates – sometimes forming bonds that will last their lifetime, sometimes having multiple partners. In addition to this, many animals, but particularly mammals, form attachments to their young whom they feed and protect from danger. They form friendships with peers and live in social groups where the prosperity of one affects that of the group and vice versa. These basic patterns of life are also recognizable within human existence, and self-confidence is central to them all.

We want the self-confidence to attract sexual partners, to develop and maintain friendships, to be an effective parent and to be successful in our role at work.

Our 'Emotion Regulation Systems'

In order to help us navigate the array of different activities that we as human beings engage in, we have systems in our brain to make us interested in and excited by achieving important goals. In addition we also have systems that make us wary and protect us if things could go wrong or we could get hurt. The compassionate mind approach uses what we know about the brain to help us understand how our emotional systems actually work. This information not only influences the therapy but is also shared with those who use it (both therapists and those receiving therapy), because if we can all truly understand ourselves better we are less prone to shame and self-criticism.

Recent research in neuroscience tells us that there are at least three types of *emotion regulation systems* (parts of our brain that work together to control and maintain our emotions). These help us achieve our key goals in life.[6] In this chapter we are going to look at the three emotional systems in some detail, but briefly they can be summarized as:

- *The threat system*: designed to help us detect and respond to threats in our lives.

- *The drive and resource acquisition system*: designed to help us detect, be interested in and take pleasure from securing important resources, enabling us to survive and prosper.

- *The contentment and soothing system*: designed to help calm and balance the other two systems (hence the term 'soothing'), giving us positive feelings of peaceful well-being and contentment.

In the compassionate mind approach we represent the three systems by the diagram opposite. Although the systems are represented by three *distinct* circles it is important to see them as continuously interacting and creating patterns in our brains. This process is represented by the arrows in the diagram. A closer examination of these systems will help you understand how emotions work, how they relate to each other, and how you can help them work in a way that allows you to build your self-confidence.

---

[6]   If you struggle with self-confidence it is likely that your *social goals* are the main group with which you'll have problems. Social goals include developing friendships and intimate relationships, taking leadership roles, becoming a parent and being valued by others.

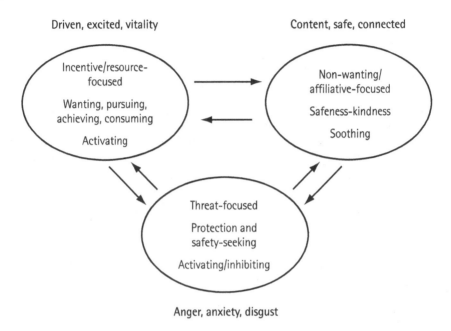

Driven, excited, vitality

Content, safe, connected

Incentive/resource-focused

Wanting, pursuing, achieving, consuming

Activating

Non-wanting/affiliative-focused

Safeness-kindness

Soothing

Threat-focused

Protection and safety-seeking

Activating/inhibiting

Anger, anxiety, disgust

Diagram 1: Three emotional regulation systems

Source: Reprinted with permission from P. Gilbert, *The Compassionate Mind* (London: Constable & Robinson, 2009).

The Threat System[7]

All living creatures need to be able to detect things that may be a danger to them – and if they live in groups and/or have offspring, they need to detect potential danger to others too. Our threat system is therefore a rapid-response centre, the first port of call for all incoming information and the system by which such information is assessed. It acts like a customs service or passport control system – only a million times faster!

The human brain, like those of other animals, has a set menu of responses that are ready to be triggered. Our three major threat-based emotions are

---

[7]   The threat system is represented by the lower circle in Diagram 1.

anxiety, anger and disgust. These are typically linked to a range of different behaviours: to freeze or run away if you're anxious; to fight or try harder if you're angry; to turn away or 'get rid of' something if you feel disgusted by it. It's easy to illustrate how quickly the threat system can be activated in us. Imagine that you are driving down a road when a cyclist suddenly appears right in front of you. There's not much time for thought. There is, however, a sudden punch in your stomach and a rush of anxiety. Alternatively, imagine you open your exam results and see an unexpected 'F'. You will immediately feel a surge of anxiety and distress. Finally, imagine you are rushing to get to work and then discover you can't find your keys, or that someone has blocked in your car. You will probably feel overcome with panic, frustration and anger.

In addition to initiating these surges of emotion, our threat system also changes the way our body works. For example, it will act to narrow and focus our attention in a crisis, and will push us towards certain behaviours in response (classically flight, fight or freeze). All of this is, of course, completely automatic, not our fault and part of our brain's basic design.

There are four important aspects to our threat system that we need to be aware of.

Our 'better safe than sorry' factory setting and the over-estimation of threat

Imagine you are trekking through the jungle and something catches your eye. The threat system will immediately respond, directing your attention to potential danger and sending a surge of anxiety through you. Your brain tells you this could be a predator. Nine times out of ten it probably isn't, but the fact is you can't afford to ignore the possibility. We call this *better safe than sorry* processing – because your brain is actually set up to overestimate threats and dangers in certain situations. We are in fact born to be 'irrational', and our tendency to 'overreact' is because our brain is designed that way.

Just to add insult to injury for many people the threat system becomes even more 'supercharged' or 'superprotective'. It's like having a smoke detector going off every time you boil an egg, or the burglar alarm ringing every time a spider moves in your house. This supercharged system is often a consequence of having lived through difficult experiences, in childhood or in later years.

The overruling of the positive

Another aspect of this system is its tendency to overrule positive feelings and events, making us focus instead on threats and negatives. Once again imagine you are trekking through the jungle and this time the thing that has caught your eye *is* a lion. Your predesigned set of responses may quickly decide that running is the best option to ensure survival. As you run you see a wonderful tree bursting with fruit, next to a river jumping with fish. Such things could feed your family for months but if you stay around to 'stock up' you are likely to become the lion's dinner. Alternatively you may not even notice the tree and the river as your attention is focused on running as fast as you can to save yourself.

In real life we are very rarely, if ever, chased by lions (well, not in the UK anyway!), but imagine walking into a room that is full of people. Nineteen out of the twenty present may look your way and smile, while one person may look over with a slightly narrowed gaze and a seemingly judgemental expression. Bang – your attention is instantly focused on that one person, you experience a rush of anxiety or anger and you find it difficult to engage with the more welcoming people around you. This is your 'better safe than sorry' factory setting at play. But what about all the people who were seemingly giving you a warm welcome? One of them could be your future best friend, another could be a potential partner. Unfortunately, you are not looking at them; your attention is on the only person who is seemingly judging you and overruling the positive.

Similarly you might have had the experience of receiving one piece of negative feedback in a sea of positive comments. Again, it is likely that your attention will go straight to the negative and you will worry about that rather than focus on all the positives.

Rumination and worry

A third aspect to the threat system, of which it is helpful to be aware, is its tendency to make you ruminate[8] on, and worry about, the negative. For example, it's Christmas and you go shopping. In nine out of ten shops the assistants are extremely helpful and you find presents that are even better than the ones you had hoped to buy. You come away feeling really pleased. Then you visit one final shop. The assistant there makes you wait while they talk to a friend, looks at you as if you were pulled through a hedge backwards, shows very little interest in helping you, sells you something that actually you don't really want, short changes you and is generally rude. So who do you talk about when you get home? You rant about that one unhelpful person who needs to be taught the rudiments of common courtesy!

Alternatively you may be planning a social gathering, inviting people you care about, some of whom you haven't seen in years. But instead of looking forward to it, you spend your time worrying whether people will come, worrying about the food and drink, about whether you will be ready in time and what the weather will be like on the day.

Simultaneous reactions pulling us in different directions

Although there are many other aspects to how the threat system works, for the purposes of this book it is helpful to reflect on this final aspect. Imagine your boss criticizes your efforts. What emotions do you feel? It may be anger associated with thoughts such as: 'How dare you criticize my work? What do you know anyway?' You may have thoughts and mental images of shouting back, punching him or taking your revenge at a later date.

---

[8]   Human beings have an ability to go 'over and over' things in their minds. Dependent upon what we focus on, this tendency can be associated with difficult emotions. When we *ruminate*, the focus is on things that have already happened. In contrast, when we *worry*, we focus on things that may happen.

There may be another part of you that feels panic and thinks, 'My work isn't good enough.' Subsequently you may want to run away, hand in your notice and/or cry. In any one situation there can be quite different and conflicting emotions and behaviours pulling us in different directions.

Just when you may be thinking this is already complicated enough, two conflicting parts of you can often react against each other. The anxious part of you may worry that your anger will get you fired, while the angry part of you may think you are being pathetic for wanting to run away, hand in your notice and/or cry. Although these conflicting emotions often occur at the same time, at others there can be a definite time lag. For example, you may be quite submissive when you are actually in a stressful situation, but then wake up in the middle of the night and think, 'Why didn't I say X? Why did I let him/her get away with it?' Or you may act very angrily in a situation and then think, 'Oh, no, I shouldn't have got angry, I've really blown it now', at a later date. It's very common for one event to result in two very different sets of emotions, behaviours and so forth, and these may well conflict with each other.

Of course all this means that we have a lot to contend with. It is an irony that the system that is set up to help us survive is exactly the same system that can make life very difficult for us.

As we will see, helping the threat system to operate more smoothly is easier said than done – but, importantly, it *is* possible.

Because our threat system often undermines us and can affect our self-confidence we will work towards recognizing when the system has been triggered and, when appropriate, aim to calm it down. Our responsibility is to let it do its job correctly and not let it run the show.

The Drive and Resource Acquisition System[9]

To survive and reproduce, animals have to do a lot more than just avoid danger. They have to find food and shelter and, of course, mates. To do

---

[9] Represented by the circle on the left in the Emotional Regulation System Diagram on p. 9.

this they need to be motivated to go out and look for things, and take pleasure in doing, achieving and acquiring.

The drive and resource acquisition system is linked to a chemical in our brain called dopamine. This is the hormone that gives us a pleasurable buzz when we achieve things. Sometimes it's a very big buzz indeed. Imagine that you have just won the Lottery and you are now worth £10 million. Assuming you're not already a millionaire, the chances are you will now have so much dopamine in your system, in reaction to the astonishing news, that you won't be able to sleep at all that night. You will be extremely excited, your head will be full of all kinds of thoughts and ideas, you'll find it difficult to wipe the smile off your face and it will certainly be a while before you will be able to settle down and watch a film with full concentration. This is your drive and resource acquisition system at play.

A system that helps us achieve and enjoy things is a good thing, except if we become over-focused on achievement to the detriment of other things. For example, many people who suffer with their self-confidence find that they seek achievement as an antidote to feeling inadequate, threatened and vulnerable. Achievement, and the positive response that it draws from others, gives them a temporary buzz and sense of self-worth. But when they are unable to keep on achieving, maybe because of age, strong competition, illness or injury, problems can arise. The primary means by which they can 'feel good' is gone, leaving a vacuum.

Some researchers, such as Jean Twenge, are concerned that modern society intentionally over-stimulates the drive and acquisition system, 'supercharging' it, so that we end up wanting more and more – more excitement, more things to do, more things to acquire – and are never quite satisfied. Powerful advertising tells us that we need more exciting computer games, faster cars, quicker telephones. They also tell us how to achieve better bodies, better skin, better hair, often pairing this with information that stimulates our threat system: 'dull, lifeless hair', 'fine lines and wrinkles'. This drives us to acquire a product or service that seemingly is the answer to all the 'problems' that have been pointed out to us. The acquisition itself gives us a buzz even if it does not give us full-bodied hair and a wrinkle-free face!

So much of present-day advertising is focused on giving us little dopamine rushes which act to stimulate our threat system. The problem is that this is not the system that leads us to feel the sense of safeness and security which is fundamental to our well-being. In addition it's not a system that really builds self-confidence because if we are driven constantly to acquire, do and achieve, the moment we find ourselves struggling or think we're *not* going to achieve something, our self-confidence collapses.

Thankfully, there is something else which enables us to feel OK about ourselves, even when things are going badly. This is the second secret to building self-confidence: self-compassion. And as we will now see, these feelings are based on a very different type of emotional regulation system.

The Contentment and Soothing System[10]

Animals enter a state of contentment and peacefulness when they have achieved what they need to achieve. This is usually when they are in a position of safety and are unlikely to come under attack. These *content states* seem to be related to the chemicals in our brain called endorphins. The state helps to promote a sense of peaceful contentment because while it is being accessed, the threat and drive systems are switched off.

When considering the primary function of the contentment and soothing system, you should bear in mind that it evolved in humans over many thousands of years, primarily as a consequence of the strong bond which exists between parent and infant. In evolutionary terms, this serves to increase the chances of the survival of the species. This system became central to what we call *attachment* and *affiliation*. Basically, the presence of the primary care giver, more usually the mother, has a calming effect on the infant and this is beneficial for both of them.

Imagine, for example, what happens when a bird flies back to feed her fledglings and sit on the nest. They become soothed and quiet. And recall the way baby penguins sit on their father's feet, cuddling up and staying

---

[10]   Represented by the circle on the right in the Emotional Regulation System Diagram on p. 9.

calm and content. They only become distressed if they lose contact with their parent. This is true of human children too. A child can be relatively calm and content until the mother or caring parent suddenly vanishes, and then it instantly becomes very distressed.

And when a child's threat system is activated, and it shows distress and anxiety, what is the thing that will calm it down and turn off the threat system? The presence of the caring parent, of course. So evolution has created a situation where the kindness and care of others has a very major impact on the regulation of our threat system, and all of this does not suddenly stop when we become adults. In fact, many scientific studies have shown that when people feel they are in caring contact with others, they are better able to deal with stress.

So from the day that you're born to the day that you die, the kindness, helpfulness and caring of others will have a huge impact on the quality of your life.

We now know that when we are born our brains contain approximately 100 billion neurons or brain cells. As we grow, the brain develops very fast. Indeed at birth it is estimated that each neuron has approximately 2,500 connections with other neurons. By the age of two or three years, each neuron has approximately 15,000 connections to other neurons. In our early years connections that are not used, or used very infrequently, disappear, while those that are regularly used multiply. So the kinds of connections that are developed and strengthened are dependent upon the kinds of experiences the baby has. If these inputs are associated with kindness, warmth and helpfulness, which serve to soothe or calm the threat system, this is what gets laid down in the baby's brain.

Later in life, the young adult will learn to use those connections to help them accept and experience positive emotions from others, such as the wider family, peers, colleagues and partners. They will also learn how to 'self-soothe', to calm and reassure themselves, and empathize with their own distress when difficult things happen.

Unfortunately, if experiences are not particularly soothing, or are actually threatening, then such positive connections may remain underdeveloped in the baby's brain. The threat system, by contrast, may become strength-ened. Consequently in adulthood the individual may find it difficult to accept and experience positive emotions in response to others, and may be more sensitive to, and perceive more, threat in their environment. They may be less able to calm and soothe themselves and therefore find it difficult to recover from life's setbacks.

It is important to stress two things at this point. Firstly, if you think that your contentment and soothing system is 'underdeveloped', it does not automatically mean that your parents or care givers are responsible for this (though at times we know this to be the case). For example, some children are born with a tendency to like lots of cuddles, and can be easily soothed, whereas others are not. Growing up, we can be affected by our siblings and peers, physical health problems, looking or being 'different' in some way, and all manner of other things that affect our experience of relationships and how we feel.

I don't wish to over-state this but it *is* the case that the human brain's development is very strongly influenced by our relationships with oth-ers, and whether those relationships go well or badly. All of this has a knock-on effect on the kind of brain we end up with.

A second very important point to stress here is that it is not too late for us to change things. We can develop or strengthen our contentment and soothing system, to help regulate our threat and drive system, at any point in our life. The key is to try and balance the systems.

Creating and Maintaining Balance – Physiotherapy for the Brain

If you wished to learn to play the piano you would put your efforts into learning the keyboard and your brain would develop accordingly. In other words, new neurons and new connections would make it possible to achieve your ambition. (Yes, contrary to popular belief, even adults make new connections and new neurons on a daily basis.) For some it may be a difficult journey but one that is ultimately worthwhile. For others it may be an enjoyable process. Similarly, if we want to enhance or maintain our well-being and self-confidence, we need to apply ourselves to it. This effort can actually *change* our brain and the way our mind works.

Because of this the compassionate mind approach often refers to this work as *physiotherapy for the brain*. However, instead of building muscle these exercises build new neural networks and pathways within the brain. Through such efforts we are able to strengthen our ability to feel differently – become more content, secure and self-confident. Once we have developed this ability, we can then work to maintain or even increase it.

Conclusions

In this chapter we have used the *three circles* to help you understand your emotional make-up a little better. Hopefully you will now be able to recognize that, as human beings, it is very easy for our very complex threat system to 'run the show'. We can also get caught up in 'feeding' our drive system, and at times this can be to our own detriment. Our contentment and soothing system, and its ability to balance the other two systems, 'keeping them in check', is key to our mental well-being.

Thankfully neurogenesis and neuroplasticity mean that we *can* change our brains and build our self-confidence. In the next chapter we will consider the typical traps we often fall into that may end up undermining our self-confidence, and we will look again at how focusing on compassion can help.

Finally, standing back from the chapter as a whole, it may help you to make a few personal observations in your journal or notebook. These may take the form of things you wish to remember or questions which this material has raised in your mind. The answers to these should become clearer as you read the rest of the book and work through the exercises it contains.

3 How and Why We Undermine Ourselves and How Compassion Can Help

As discussed in Chapter 1, we human beings have a whole range of ways in which we can undermine our own self-confidence! Most people will be able to identify with each of these to a greater or lesser extent. However, as people vary in the degree to which they undermine themselves, so too does the toll this takes on them.

The biggest culprits for self-undermining are:

- Shame

- Over-striving and perfectionism

- Self-criticism

Too much versus too little information

For some individuals the detail I will go into here will be exactly what they need in order to truly understand themselves better. Others may find this wealth of information counter productive, especially when they wish to start 'doing' something. It is worth noting, however, that understanding ourselves *is* a key part of 'doing' as it helps counteract some of the ways in which we habitually undermine ourselves.

Those who would like more information on shame and self-undermining than is outlined in this chapter will find a further reading list at the end of the book.

In this chapter we are going to look at how we habitually undermine ourselves. Simply being able to recognize these habits in yourself can be a huge step forward towards addressing them and changing things for the better.

At the end of this chapter we will look at a few examples which illustrate how focusing on self-compassion instead of self-criticism can help to build self-confidence.

Shame and How it Undermines Our Self-confidence

Shame can prevent us from building our self-confidence because it rarely, if ever, allows us to let people 'in'. We may hide behind a mask or an image we wish to portray to others, and this decreases the likelihood of our ever receiving the validation we need. It may be helpful therefore to examine shame, in all its guises, in more detail.

The power of shame

Most of us have a sense of what we mean by shame. It is related to feeling bad about ourselves, and in some way feeling that other people see us as inadequate, inferior or incompetent. To help you understand the extent to which shame can affect you, I would like you to try the brief exercise below.

Exercise 1: How shame affects your mind and body

Just for a moment think back to a time when you felt ashamed. Try not to bring to mind anything too major; we simply want to touch briefly on the feeling.

Once you have managed to connect with that experience of shame, spend a little time asking yourself the questions below. If you find it difficult to answer them, briefly revisit the memory and try once more to give some answers.

- How did shame feel in your body? For example, did you notice a sensation as if your heart were sinking or an unusual feeling in your stomach? Did you feel hot or maybe experience an increase in your heart rate?

- What kind of thoughts went through your mind about yourself and about what other people might be thinking of you?

- What emotions did you feel? Perhaps you felt anxious or angry, maybe confused or simply paralyzed, finding it difficult to think or feel anything.

- What did you want to do? Did you want to run away, curl into a ball or lash out?

Now, having answered each of these questions, take a few minutes to let the experience fade from your mind and body.[11]

By completing this simple exercise you will become more aware that when you experience shame it can result in a whole array of different reactions. These include physical sensations, certain types of emotions and thoughts, as well as the urge to react in various ways. Shame typically involves feeling exposed in some way, paired with the experience of feeling flawed, inadequate or bad.

Often it silences us; our head goes down and we want to creep away, stay in the background. However, this is not always the case. Sometimes when people feel shame, rather than feeling inferior and submissive, they can react with aggression and feel the urge to fight back. Although we are not going to explore the problem of anger specifically here, those who identify with this may find Russell Kolts' book in this series, *The Compassionate Mind Approach to Managing Your Anger*, of interest.

---

[11]   If a feeling of unease or heightened emotion remains after you have carried out this exercise or any in the book it may be helpful to you to recall a recent time when you have felt content and comfortable, maybe on your own or with someone else, and let this image fill your mind and body.

Understanding how shame works in us, and what we can do about it, are two very important steps on the way to developing self-confidence. Let's look at this in more detail.

Compassion-focused therapist Professor Paul Gilbert has spent a long time researching shame and points out that it has three types of focus. He has named these:

- Reflected shame

- External shame

- Internal shame

We are now going to look at each of these in turn. As you will see, it is likely that internal and external shame are most closely associated with the undermining of self-confidence, and for this reason we will focus most strongly on these two categories of shame in this book.

The origins of Compassion Focused Therapy (CFT)

CFT was originally developed specifically for people who experience high levels of shame. Therapists and researchers, as well as those experiencing such difficulties, had observed that more traditional forms of therapy were not meeting their needs. People who experience shame have often experienced a number of difficulties in their early lives, maybe in the family context or at school. It is understandable that, given such experiences, it can be difficult for people to feel safe in the world, safe in the therapy, or even to like themselves much. This can impact on an individual's efforts to build self-confidence.

Reflected shame

Reflected shame is what *we* may feel in response to *other* people's actions; it is not about us directly. Alternatively, it is the shame *other* people feel because of *our* actions. For example, we may feel reflected shame because a member of our family has done a particular thing that is deemed 'shameful'.

This form of shame has been looked at within certain cultural communities by Jasvinder Sanghera. In her book *Shame*, Jasvinder drew on her own background and explored the experiences of a subsection of Asian women who are forced into arranged marriages. The experience of reflected shame can be so serious in some cultures that it may lead to so-called honour killing of those deemed to have brought shame on their families.

The experience of reflected shame can also be less serious and, for some of us, border more on embarrassment, especially after some time has passed. Many parents have squirmed when their child points out something about another person (usually within earshot!), maybe about their size, their hair colour, their wrinkles, or any other characteristics. We may apologize, raise our eyes or laugh awkwardly, but even when we know their words are totally innocent we still feel reflected shame at that moment, as though our child's actions are a reflection on us. It's only later, when the shame turns into embarrassment, that we may be able to laugh at the situation with a friend or partner.

Alternatively, for those of you who, like me, have a dog, reflected shame is the experience you have when it decides to go to the toilet in an inappropriate place or sniffs another dog where you know it will (but wish it wouldn't). It is amazing how, at that moment, I can feel shame about what my dog is doing – as if his behaviour is a reflection on me!

Reflected shame is considered to serve a number of functions. You may wish to consider reading Jasvinder Sanghera's book, or there are a number of titles by Paul Gilbert if you wish to study this area further. More information can be found in the Further Reading section at the end of this book (page 261).

External shame

External shame is associated with the idea that other people are thinking negatively about us. Maybe your boss criticizes your work and you feel belittled in his or her eyes. Maybe having put on weight, or due to another aspect of your appearance, you think other people are judging you negatively.

Upon feeling that someone is viewing us negatively, we may alter our behaviour. For example, we may become very submissive at work or even stop going out. We may dress to disguise a perceived flaw, become over-apologetic or maybe lash out. External shame is the sense we have of *how we exist in the minds of others,* and some of us worry about this a great deal. The more we worry about the way other people judge us and feel about us, the more this can work to undermine our own self-confidence.

But why do we worry about what other people feel and think about us? Well, there are a couple of very good reasons for this.

First, in order for our contentment and soothing system (see Chapter 2) to develop, we need the kindness and caring of others. We also need to make, initially basic, but later more complex, judgements about who is safe and who is not. Human beings have an in-built mechanism that motivates us to look at others and wonder, 'What are they thinking about or feeling towards me?' and, ultimately, 'Whom can I trust?' In childhood, and into adulthood, we hopefully develop the capacity to *self-regulate,* to soothe or reassure ourselves in the face of life's knocks. This obviously helps us to secure our place in the world, but it is still vitally important for us to be able to think about what is going on in the minds of other people.

Our ability to cope with external shame, or the possibility that others may not think as highly of us as we'd like them to, often comes down to our own self-confidence and ability to self-regulate. In summary, we human beings are predestined to spend time trying to work out what other people think of us. If we have had difficult experiences, usually in childhood but maybe after that, we are more sensitive to threat from others. Working to develop our contentment and soothing system can help us regulate or 'tone down' the sense of threat, but it can also give us self-confidence in our ability to deal with such situations. The more self-confident we feel within ourselves, the easier it is to cope when things aren't quite as we would like them to be.

Second, Paul Gilbert points out that the experience of external shame alerts us to the possibility of being rejected in some way. It also potentially guides us to different behaviours that may make it more likely we are accepted and protected by those around us. If others see us nega-tively then they are less likely to be our friends, want to interact with us or support us when times are hard. If, on the other hand, they feel good about us and like us then it is more likely they will want to be our friends and help us. So in a way external shame warns us about how we exist in the minds of others, which has had important implications initially for our survival and, in more recent times, for our well-being also.

Humans are highly motivated to seek the praise and approval of others, and have an inherent need to belong and to share. Consequently it really hurts if we feel there are things about us that will devalue us in other people's eyes or detract from our endeavours.

It is important to recognize that we all like to feel valued and wanted by those around us. There is no shame in this. It is a deep-rooted trait that has proved highly significant in evolutionary terms. Approval from others helps us feel safe in the world; part of the group. However, if we feel bad about ourselves, we may feel under more scrutiny from others, perceive more social threat than is warranted, and this in turn may mean that we 'over-strive' to be accepted. As we will see later, this 'over-striving' can itself cause us problems.

Internal shame

The final kind of shame is internal, where our attention is fixed upon our-selves, or how we think and feel about ourselves. Sometimes there appears to be consistency between what other people seem to feel and think about us and how we view ourselves, whilst at other times people may be very complimentary to us while our own judgements are much more negative.

For example, if we are subtly bullied in our social group, and the butt of many of the jokes, we can start to think that what people are saying is true and begin to feel the same way about ourselves. As a result we may feel both external and internal shame. However, in another scenario, we may find that despite everyone commenting favourably on our work and stating that we are a good friend or partner, we feel very different about ourselves. We still feel internal shame, as though there is something wrong with us. Then, because what people say is inconsistent with the way we view ourselves, we may start to think 'They're only saying that', 'If they really knew me they wouldn't like me', or 'They are lulling me into a false sense of security'.

Internal shame is probably one of the biggest underminers of self-confidence there is. And one of the most important aspects of internal shame is *self-criticism*, which we will discuss later in this chapter.

But whether it is reflected, external or internal shame, or a blend of all three, shame undermines our self-confidence because while suffering from it we rarely, if ever, let people see the true person underneath. We hide behind an image we wish to promote to others and so decrease the likelihood of our ever being valued for the person we really are. It is like building a house with no foundations – we may achieve great things, but we constantly undermine our own success by attributing it not to ourselves but to other factors. The resulting feeling of instability is like living permanently with the threat of our house falling down around our ears.

How Over-striving and Perfectionism Can Undermine Our Self-confidence

In this next section we will look at over-striving and perfectionism. As you will see, these two areas overlap with those outlined above. However, in an effort to understand and therefore be kinder to yourself, it can be helpful to consider different ways of viewing things in the hope that something will resonate for you.

Over-striving

One way in which we often try and deal with external shame is to try and *prove ourselves* to other people. Psychologists have researched how this desire to prove ourselves can instead undermine our self-confidence.

Over fifty years ago researchers into human motivation pointed out that

we can be motivated to achieve things in different ways, and they catego-
rized achievement in the following two subsections:

1. Value achievers

People in this group derive pleasure from doing things because they
feel value in the achievement *itself.* This may include swimming a mile,
climbing a mountain, passing exams or taking up a particular career.
Even small achievements give them pleasure.

2. Need achievers

This group, who seem similarly motivated to swim the mile, climb the
mountain, pass exams and so on, seem to derive less pleasure from the
achievement itself. By contrast they derive pleasure mostly from the
applause, approval and accolades that accompany the achievement.
Indeed, if the activity does not bring any such accolades or approval,
they quickly stop doing it. These people are termed *need achievers* because
they need achievement as a means of gaining approval and feeling valued by others. Notice how the two approaches can outwardly look quite
similar, but are not.

It is important that we start to think carefully about our goals and values,
and why we do exactly what we do. There is nothing wrong with being
a need achiever and wanting the approval of others, but we've got to be
careful as this approach to life can leave us open to disappointment, is
less predictable, and can work to undermine self-confidence. Of course
most of us are a blend of value and need achievers, most of the time, but
people who struggle with self-confidence tend to be more on the need-
achiever side of things.

In time, researchers looked at motivation in slightly different ways.
Benjamin Dykman, for example, suggested there are two main motivations behind achievement. These are:

1. Growth seeking

Growth seekers enjoy challenges and their ability to learn. As such, they
mature through positively learning by their mistakes. If you have this

attitude to life then very clearly you're going to be continually building your self-confidence because you are going to be learning how to deal with mistakes and constantly getting better at things.

2. Validation seeking

Similar to *need achievers* outlined above, Dykman used the term *validation seekers* to describe individuals who feel under constant pressure to prove themselves as likeable and acceptable to others, suggesting that validation seeking develops in childhoods where children are constantly uncertain of being loved and valued. Alternatively, validation seekers may come from families where others were perfectionists and much was expected of them. We can see how this scenario developed for Kelly.

Kelly's story

Kelly came from a family where both parents were quite demanding and critical of her. She constantly felt she had to live up to their expectations and prove herself to them. They were not unkind to her, nor were they lacking in some degree of affection, though they were not a family who demonstrated this in any way.

Kelly grew up with a sense of needing constantly to strive to prove herself and a nagging sense of not being 'good enough'. In fact, she reported that she only felt OK with herself when she had succeeded at something that other people placed value on (and even this was short-lived). Although to others her self-confidence *seemed* adequate, in certain areas it was actually quite fragile as Kelly felt everything could come tumbling down around her at any moment if she took her eye off the ball.

Perfectionism

Although perfectionism can be helpful at certain times and in certain aspects of our lives, it can also undermine our self-confidence. This is thought to be down to certain forms of perfectionism and, once again, if you identify with this trait, it may be important to think about which one applies to you.

In a series of studies psychologist David Dunkley and colleagues demonstrated that there are at least two types of perfectionism that look the same but are very different. They are as follows:

1. High standards for the sake of the standards themselves

You want an individual with this sort of perfectionism to be your brain surgeon because he/she is very careful and his/her standards are exacting. These people are highly motivated and gain pleasure from perfection itself.

2. High standards for the sake of 'evaluative concerns'

These individuals are frightened of making mistakes, frightened of rejection and frightened of being shamed. Dunkley and colleagues found that people who were perfectionistic because they were concerned about what other people thought were much more vulnerable to all kinds of mental health difficulties.[12]

It's not just as a consequence of our family environment that such concerns arise. Children who are vulnerable to bullying or feeling marginalized at school, because, for example, they are not quite so good at sports or look a certain way, can sometimes develop this great need to prove themselves in order to be included. If we wish to build our self-confidence it is helpful for us to stop trying to prove ourselves and instead make active choices about the changes it may be helpful for us to make. While wanting to prove ourselves to others, and be approved of, is absolutely essential to being human (imagine people who didn't care what other people thought of them), the most important thing is to achieve balance.

---

[12]   Paul Gilbert and colleagues have also looked at the link between such factors and mental health problems, and have shown that when we strive to avoid inferiority (which is different from seeking superiority), we often do so because we are frightened of being excluded and rejected. This in turn sets us up for problems with anxiety and depression.

If the balance swings too far in favour of needing to prove yourself, rather than enjoying your achievements and learning from your mistakes, you will get into difficulties. High levels of fear or concern about what other people might think can manifest themselves in all kinds of difficulties, from shyness to social anxiety and even depression.

Lynne Henderson has written a book on shyness and social anxiety in the Compassionate Mind series: *Improving Social Confidence and Reducing Shyness Using Compassion Focused Therapy*. You may want to take a look at it if this seems to be a particular problem for you. In her book she deals primarily with *social* confidence whereas here we are looking more at self-confidence.

Self-criticism and How it Undermines Our Self-confidence

Self-criticism is very easy to misunderstand. It can at times be helpful and yet at others it can undermine our self-confidence. The key to understanding whether it is helpful or not for you is to notice the emotions and motivations that accompany it. To help explore what emotions and motivations are associated with your own self-criticism grab a pen or pencil and your notebook or journal and work through Exercise 2 below. The exercise may be associated with difficult emotions so you may wish to try it only briefly.

Exercise 2: Identifying your self-critic

Think back to a recent occasion when you were critical of yourself and your efforts. Nothing too major because you just want to *glimpse* the critical part of yourself. The situation may focus on something you found difficult at work, a time when you lost your keys or wallet or maybe when you made some form of mistake.

Once you are able to bring a situation to mind, imagine that the self-critical part of you could be viewed as a person. Now read through the following questions and jot down the answers in the space provided or in your journal/notebook.

Part 1

1. If your self-critical thoughts took on the appearance of an actual person, what would they look like?

2. What would their facial expression be?

3. Are they physically big or small in comparison to you?

4. What is their tone of voice like?

5. If you can imagine their body, what is their posture and body like?

6. What emotions are they directing your way?

7. Do they remind you of anyone?

Part 2

Now you have completed the imagery part of this exercise it's time for reflection.

What have you discovered?

Having gone through each section, take a few minutes to let the experience fade from your mind and body.[13]

Often when we look in detail at the self-critical part of ourselves we find that it is associated with feelings of frustration, contempt and anger. We may find that the self-critical part is either a figure that looms large or a little gremlin that wags its finger in constant reproof. Often their tone of voice is hostile and, for some, this exercise evokes memories or images of someone from the past, someone who was critical of us and our efforts.

Discoveries other people have made from this exercise:

For many people the exercise illustrates that their own self-critic is a bully. The image they generate may be someone from the past or an amalgamation of people. Others realize it is unlikely such a critic would be helpful to them as they actually feel immobilized in their presence.

So why do we engage in self-criticism?

In order to answer this I would like you to try a further exercise.

---

[13]   If a feeling of unease or heightened emotion remains after you have engaged in this exercise it may be helpful now to recall a recent time when you have felt content and comfortable, maybe on your own or with someone else, and let this image fill your mind and body.

Exercise 3: Recognizing the fears we may have about letting go of self-criticism and the benefits we attribute to it

For a moment, just imagine that we can take away your self-criticism. What are your greatest fears about giving it up?

What do you think might happen?

When you look at your self-critic and you see the emotions coming back to you from it, to what extent do you think it genuinely had your best interests at heart?

Does it really care about you and take great joy in seeing you flourish, do well and be happy?

If your self-critic does have your best interests at heart, is it going about things in the right way?

What have you discovered?

Having answered each of the questions, take a few minutes to let the experience fade from your mind and body.

It is likely that you have fears associated with letting go of your self-criticism. Yet this is most probably tinged with frustration and disappointment, anger or even contempt. As such, it's probably not the best part of you to help build your self-confidence. In actual fact it is more likely to drag you down and undermine both you and your efforts.

Learning from mistakes is very important, but we have a much better chance of doing this, and doing it in a sustained way, if we go about it by building and nurturing our self-confidence rather than undermining ourselves with self-criticism, frustration and contempt.

To illustrate this point further it may be helpful to engage in the following exercise.

Exercise 4: Choosing who is best placed to guide you in the building of your self-confidence

Read the following scenario and imagine yourself into it.

You have a child for whom you care greatly. When you enrol the child at school there are two parallel classes for your son's or daughter's age group and you have a choice between the different classes and their teachers. You visit one class and the first teacher tells you they are going to help your child to improve by acting quickly to correct their mistakes. This will result in, for example, having something taken away from them or sitting at the front of the class so that they learn not to make the same mistake twice. While the teacher is relaying this information to you, a child in the class spills a drink across the table and on to the floor. Immediately the teacher notices and shouts at them in a stern voice to be more careful, telling them to clear up the mess they have made and *never* to be so clumsy again. To reinforce this message the child is given twenty lines to write out. The teacher whispers in your ear: 'If they learn that bad things happen after mistakes, they quickly learn not to make them.'

On leaving you go straight to the other class. By contrast the second teacher tells you that they feel it is very important for children to profit by their mistakes, to be open about them, curious about how they came about, and to learn how they can prevent them in the future. As you are speaking a child's knife and fork clatter to the floor (both visits were occurring at lunchtime!). The second teacher quickly approaches the child, squats down next to him, and in a gentle and inquisitive voice says, 'What happened?' 'I was putting my hand up for second helpings and my elbow caught my knife, and that caught my fork and . . .' 'John, given that this happened, what do you need to remember the next time you want to put your hand up for seconds?' And so the conversation between child and teacher continues for a little while in this gentle manner.

Which teacher would you choose for your child?

If the answer is the second teacher, take a moment to reflect why are you always sending yourself to the first?

Having answered each of the questions above, take a few minutes to let the impact of the experience fade from your mind.

'We have to learn to be our own best friends because we fall too easily into the trap of being our own worst enemies'

– Roderick Thorp, *Rainbow Drive*

You may decide that making such choices is easy when things are going relatively well, but what about when things are difficult and you need to have courage? In answer to this, briefly imagine that you are going into a burning house. Who would you like to give you cover and support as you go in? Someone who is reassuring and encouraging or someone who is quick to criticize and shout (making you more anxious) when you get into difficulties? It's a no-brainer. When things get tough you need a friend by your side. This is basically the essence of Compassion Focused Therapy. We build self-confidence by learning how to become a good friend to ourselves. This means being neither too critical (or in extreme cases tearing ourselves to bits) nor too passive, always saying 'There, there . . . poor you'. A good friend will have your best interests at heart. They will be sympathetic to all that life throws at you but will encourage you and be your cheerleader when you have something you need to face. Indeed, what we are going to do throughout this book is learn how to develop self-compassion, which brings support and encouragement, together with qualities such as strength, empathy and non-judgement.

Paul Gilbert, in his book *The Compassionate Mind*, makes the distinction between shame-based self-criticism (maybe what you do at the moment) and compassionate self-correction, and uses the table on page 37 to help us compare the two.

So compassionate self-correction (or, the term I personally use 'compassionate self-adjustments') wins hands down every time.

Hope in the Shape of Our Brain's *Amazing* Abilities

If you're still not convinced of the need to address our habit of undermining ourselves and to develop self-compassion instead, hopefully the following section will help consolidate the idea. In Compassion Focused Therapy we discuss how, in everyday life, thoughts and images can influence the way our brains and bodies work. This can be beneficial in helping us to make informed decisions or to take more control over what we think and imagine.

Table 1: Distinguishing between shame-based self-criticism and compassionate self-correction

Shame-based self-criticism	Compassionate self-correction
• Focuses on the desire to condemn and punish	• Focuses on the desire to improve
• Punishes past errors and is often backward-looking	• Emphasizes growth and enhancement
• Is given with anger, frustration contempt, disappointment	• Is forward-looking
• Concentrates on deficits and fear of exposure	• Is given with encouragement, support, kindness
• Focuses on a global sense of self	• Builds on positives (e.g. seeing what you did well and then considering learning points)
• Includes a high fear of failure	• Focuses on attributes and specific qualities of self
• Increases chances of avoidance and withdrawal.	• Emphasizes hope for success
	• Increases the chances of engaging.
Consider example of critical teacher with a child who is struggling.	Consider example of encouraging, supportive teacher with a child who is struggling.
For transgression	*For transgression*
• Shame, avoidance, fear	• Guilt, engaging
• Heart sinks, lowered mood	• Sorrow, remorse
• Aggression.	• Reparation.

Reprinted with permission from P. Gilbert, *The Compassionate Mind* (London: Constable & Robinson, 2009).

How our brains respond to stimulus

Imagine that you are very hungry and you see a wonderful plate of food or smell amazing scents coming from the kitchen. What happens to your saliva and stomach acids? They get going, don't they? This is because the sight and smell of the food stimulate an area of your brain called the *hypothalamus* and its job is to prepare your body for eating. But supposing it's late at night and maybe all the shops are closed, or you have no money, so you just sit and find yourself *fantasizing* about a lovely meal to satisfy your hunger. What happens to your saliva and stomach acids now? They get going in exactly the same way, don't they? Isn't that interesting? Just the *image* and the *thought* of food can stimulate the same area to release acids into your stomach because your brain thinks you're about to eat.

Let's think about another situation. What happens if you go for a night out and meet someone you find really attractive? You flirt with each other and towards the end of the evening they lean in towards you to kiss you. (You can tell a female is writing this, can't you!) In this situation you are likely to become aroused. Signals will go straight to your brain and stimulate an area called the *pituitary gland* which will release hormones into your body and those will cause arousal. But here is the important part – supposing you simply *imagine* all of this happening. What happens in your body then? What is interesting is that human beings can derive arousal simply through deliberately created *mental imagery*, and this stimulates the pituitary gland in exactly the same way as if the imaginary scenario were *really* happening. The point here is that the different images *you create* in your head can stimulate different areas in your body. When you *imagine* a meal you are stimulating your hypothalamus; when you *imagine* things that are sexually arousing you are stimulating your pituitary gland.

It's very clear that in these everyday situations our thoughts and mental imagery can actually have a major effect on our bodies. We all know this, of course, but often don't really see the full implications – and these are huge.

If you experience bullying at school or at work, it is likely that this will activate your threat system. You may experience anxiety, anger or sadness. You may feel the urge to fight, run, or may freeze. You may even experience all of these feelings at once.

But what happens when, instead of *being* bullied by someone else, we bully and criticize *ourselves*, taunt ourselves with things we are unhappy with or that make us feel ashamed? What happens when we are constantly unkind, critical and harsh towards ourselves and let our self-critical part get the upper hand and run the show? What part of the brain are we stimulating then? These thoughts, images and memories are going to stimulate the threat system, over and over, as if those things are constantly recurring. And going back to the three-circle model that we saw in Chapter 2, you'll see that if you continually stimulate the threat system with certain internal thoughts, memories and imagery, it will become out of balance.

So although it can seem that the critical part of ourselves has our best interests at heart, it actually stimulates the threat system over and over again. This then triggers a further layer of emotions, narrowing our attention and predisposing us towards predesigned responses such as fight, flight or freeze. How can this scenario ever build self-confidence? It can only undermine it.

As we have seen previously, if we grow up in and experience a nurturing environment we are more likely to feel a sense of contentment. But what happens if we *learn* how to be kind and supportive to ourselves? In this new frame of mind, what would happen if we tried to understand why we experienced difficulties?

Imagine what would happen if you committed yourself to really building your self-confidence by generating a friendly voice in your head that was always supportive of you. A voice that was strong and instilled courage into you with which to face life's difficulties. This would build and maintain your contentment and soothing system, and help to bring emotional balance. Maybe in this mindset you might also feel encouraged and inspired, and this would also stimulate your drive system in a helpful way. Diagram 2 on page 40 may help to summarize this.

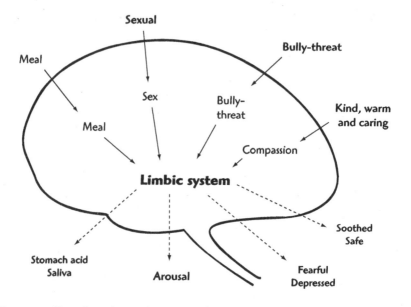

Diagram 2: How thoughts and imagery affect our brains and bodies

Source: Reprinted with permission from P. Gilbert, *The Compassionate Mind* (London: Constable & Robinson, 2009).

How we speak to ourselves is extremely important

From a scientific perspective, Paul Gilbert and colleagues have looked at what happens in the brain when we are kind and self-reassuring, in contrast to being self-critical. They have found evidence that self-reassurance and self-criticism stimulate quite different systems in our brains. This therefore suggests that the tone we use to speak to ourselves is very important.

Conclusions

If we can gain a greater understanding of the way our mind works, and a better awareness of the traps we fall into, we can then learn to implement more helpful strategies: ones that will increase rather than knock our self-confidence. Building self-confidence begins with recognizing what we're doing to ourselves, acknowledging that problems with self-confidence are not our fault but arise from the way our brains are designed, and then making a commitment to change things for the better.

The rest of this book is going to be helping you do exactly that – build your self-confidence by fostering a better relationship with yourself. Following this path will help you gain the strength and courage needed to face, engage with and address the difficulties you may have in your life rather than avoid them.

4 Making Sense of Your Experiences

In Chapters 1 to 3 we saw that self-confidence is something you need to build and maintain, *not* something you are either born with or without. We then went on to look at self-confidence from an evolutionary perspective, and at examples of the ways in which we can often undermine ourselves and therefore stunt the development of self-confidence. Finally we looked at how developing compassion can help.

In this chapter you will find some exercises that have been specifically designed to help you develop a compassionate understanding of your own difficulties. This may help to counteract any self-undermining and provide a platform on which to build your self-confidence. The exercises involve:

- Understanding what has influenced you

- Recognizing your key concerns and fears

- Noting your coping strategies, why you may adopt them, and their unintended consequences

- Developing your own formulation

- Making sense of things

It is worth noting that, for some, undertaking the exercises within this chapter can be an emotional experience. The exercises can spotlight difficult things that have happened in the past and give rise to some troubling shoulds, shouldn'ts and if onlys. You may find that you slip into self-criticism and feel emotions such as sadness, anger, anxiety or maybe shame. Later in this book we will find ways of dealing with these, but the first step is to understand the origins of the difficulties you may be experiencing, how they affect you and how this in turn impacts on your self-confidence.

At the end of the chapter we will read Andy's story and look at his personal formulation. This should give you an idea of how others have gained an understanding of the influences brought to bear on them, the coping strategies adopted – and their unintended consequences.

Our Influences: Nature and Nurture

Most people agree that we are the product of *both* nature and nurture. In other words, a combination of our biology (nature) and our experiences (nurture) influences who we are.

Let's look at this in a bit more detail. First, our genes can predispose us to a certain temperament; they can give us the capacity to reach a particular level of academic or emotional intelligence. Genes influence the way we look and can predispose us to certain physical health difficulties. Secondly, our genes and biology are influenced and shaped by the environment we find ourselves in. This begins from the moment we are conceived and can include experiencing certain life events such as moving schools, bereavement and problematic relationships with our peers, influences exerted by our family environment such as the effect brothers and sisters may have on us, how we are parented and the kind of place we live in. We are also affected by society in general, such as how our culture is viewed, our sexual orientation or our religious beliefs.

Exercise 5: Noting what has influenced you

An infinite number of things shape our lives, but listed below in worksheet 1 are some common ones that can be associated with difficulties with self-confidence. Some of them may apply to you, others may not. Read through the list and, if you find something that you recognize, place a tick next to it or write it down in your notebook.

You may find this hard to do on your first attempt. It may be helpful to consider your life in separate periods of time and in different environments. For example, what may have influenced you up to the point of starting primary school? What about the time at each school you attended? At that time what was affecting you at home, at school and in other areas of your life? And so forth.

It is quite likely that the list in the worksheet below will not cover everything that has had, and/or still has, an influence on your self-confidence. Further space is provided at the bottom of the table where you may add any other experiences you have thought of that affected your self-confidence.

Worksheet 1 : Influences on me

Growing up around people who lacked self-confidence
Growing up around people who were seemingly 'good at everything' when I found myself to be less so
Love and affection being seemingly dependent on success
Being around people who were self-critical and/or critical of *me*
Experiencing little love and/or affection
Being naturally more introverted or shy
Bereavements

Loss of key friendships – due to moving house, moving school or both
Having physical difficulties
Unusual experiences, such as seeing or hearing things other people don't seem to see or hear
Having difficulties such as dyslexia, dyspraxia, dyscalculia, making learning difficult
Experiencing bullying or indifference from my peers or siblings
Difficult relationships – be it friendships or sexual relationships
Traumatic events such as physical, sexual or emotional abuse, being the victim of crime or being involved in some form of accident
Experiencing difficult teaching styles
Looking 'different' from other people
Issues related to my sexuality or identity
Other influences on me:

Further thoughts about the things that influence us

It is worth noting that although you are currently being encouraged to reflect on difficult times, it is likely that in your life and/or current situation there have also been some positive influences and experiences that have been beneficial to or protective of you. These may be easy for you to recall, or they may be more difficult because of low mood or high levels of anxiety which 'cloud the picture'. For some of us, unfortunately, there may be a simple lack of such positive influences and experiences.

To complicate things further, some influences and experiences associated with difficulties in self-confidence may arise from scenarios that are not obviously problematic. Here are a few examples:

- It is likely that all parents have a mixture of positive and negative influences on their children.

- Self-confident siblings can be fun to be around and can help us do things, but they can also prevent us building our own self-confidence when they do everything for us. We don't learn that we can do things for ourselves.

- A very close family, with whom we do everything, may be a great environment to grow up in, but it may also mean that we have little experience of doing things outside the immediate family other than at school, and this can prevent aspects of our self-confidence from developing.

- Physical health problems, may, in some areas of our lives, restrict us, result in pain and discomfort, and cause other problems. However, they may also give us a sense of identity with other people who experience similar problems and in certain situations may result in us feeling 'special'.

- Being a twin may be a very special experience but it may mean we are always judged against our sibling. For example, people may ask 'Which is the naughty one?' or 'Which is the self-confident one?' and you may be labelled as such. Alternatively you may have the experience of always being viewed as 'the same' as your sibling. Being a twin can also prevent other friendships from developing.

- Being the eldest child may mean you spent more time individually with your parents in your early years, you might have been given additional responsiblities, there may be more photos of you, and more might have been made of such events as your first day at school. Being the eldest can also mean, however, that you have to be more 'grown up' than your siblings when they were the same age, and the arrival of younger siblings meant you felt you had to share your parents more. In a similar way, being a middle or youngest child can also have both pluses and negatives.

Key Concerns and Fears

It is understandable that based on our experiences we may develop key concerns or fears. These then drive or influence our behaviour, our emotions, our thinking and focus of attention as well as our physiology. These concerns or fears can be separated into two categories:

- Concerns and fears relating to, or about, our *external world*, such as what people may think of us or how they may behave towards us.

- Concerns and fears relating to, or about, our *internal world*, such as what we think about ourselves.

Exercise 6: Recognizing your key concerns and fears

Listed in worksheet 2 (pages 49–50) are a number of common concerns and fears that can be linked to difficulties with self-confidence. Some of them may apply to you, others may not. Read through the list and place a tick next to the ones that you have experienced or currently identify with. Alternatively you may wish to jot them down in your notebook.

Once again, because it is impossible to cover all of the concerns and fears people have, things may come to your mind that are not listed. If this is the case please use the space provided to jot down your own thoughts.

Alternatively you may find that although you identify with one of the concerns or fears, you would word things differently. If this is the case, use your own words to describe how it applies to you.

Things may not initially spring to mind or it may be difficult to recall former fears and concerns because you are presently in a different frame of mind. It may be helpful to spend a little time reflecting on this in the following ways:

- Think back to difficult periods in your life, maybe using the points you identified with in the previous exercise as a prompt.

- Think about recent occasions when you have experienced anxiety, sadness or anger. What were the concerns or fears that were uppermost in your mind at that time?

Things that we can easily become fearful of:

It is worth noting that as a consequence of our evolution we are *programmed* to be wary or scared of certain harmful things so as to ensure the survival of the species. Fears that are quick to develop in us include fear of heights, fear of things that move erratically such as spiders, fear of confined spaces and the dark. In addition, because we are a social species, we are also primed to be wary or scared of any degree of social threat. This may involve becoming wary when someone appears to be evaluating us negatively or looks angry. As a consequence we constantly monitor and react to potential threats from others. This evolutionary *wiring* helps us 'stay part of the group', from which we derive strength and protection. It is therefore not surprising that what underpins many of the feelings and concerns are fears about negative judgement from others, as this could lead to social isolation.

Worksheet 2 : Key concerns and fears

Fears and concerns relating to my external world
People will think badly of me or judge me
People will behave negatively towards me (verbally, physically, etc.)
Others will reject me
I will be isolated from people
Other fears and concerns I have in relation to my external world:

Worksheet 2 : Key concerns and fears (continued)

Fears and concerns relating to my internal world
My emotions will get the better of me or are dangerous
I will not be able to or cannot control my actions
The thoughts and mental images I have are dangerous
There is something wrong with me – physically or mentally
Other fears and concerns I have in relation to my internal world:

Coping Strategies and Their Consequences

A combination of influences and experiences can lead us to develop certain concerns and fears. It is these that can drive us towards protective or coping strategies that are meant to help us. While some strategies appear to be intentional choices, others seem more automatic. Although designed to be helpful to us, many of the things we do have unfortunate unintended consequences or drawbacks. We will look at these in the next exercise.

Exercise 7: Noting your coping strategies, why you may adopt them, and their unintended consequences

Read through the categories listed in worksheet 3 (pages 52–57) and put a tick against those that apply to you. It is likely that you will recognize that you do certain things, but the reasons why you do them (their 'intended function'), or their unintended consequences or drawbacks, may not be listed. For this reason there is space provided to make further notes against each example. You may also have other coping strategies that are not listed. As with the previous worksheets there is space for you to make a note of these at the bottom of the sheet.

Of course we all feel or do many of these things from time to time. Problems occur when we feel or do them *to excess*.

In addition to the *specific* unintended consequences or drawbacks outlined above, many of the strategies listed can cause more *universal* problems, such as putting strain on our close relationships. More importantly, they can also prevent us from building our self-confidence because we tend to attribute any success to the strategies themselves, and the failures to ourselves alone. This often reinforces our key concerns and fears, creating a vicious cycle – sad and frustrating, isn't it?

Worksheet 3 : Intended and unintended consequences of your coping strategies

Coping strategy	Intended consequence	Possible unintended consequences or drawbacks
Being as others want	Avoid rejection Avoid conflict Keep people happy	Feelings of resentment towards other people Own needs are not met Exhausting
Keep people at arm's length	Avoid rejection/ disappointment Avoid conflict	Isolating Low mood Anxiety
Always 'putting a happy or brave face on'/wearing a 'mask'	Avoid rejection/ disappointment	Exhausting No one knows the true you Prevents a feeling of true acceptance from others

Coping strategy	Intended consequence	Possible unintended consequences or drawbacks
Defer to or rely on others	Avoid failure Avoid anxiety	Feelings of resentment Prevents own skills developing
Settling for things that are not ideal – 'making do'	Prevents disappointment	Resentment Conflict Things become mediocre
Avoid certain situations such as interviews, dates, public speaking	Reduce chance of disappointment/rejection Avoid anxiety and potential low mood if things don't go right	Not reaching personal goals Lack of opportunity to experience a sense of achievement
Only going certain places or doing certain things with particular people	Decrease anxiety Gives greater sense of predictability	Resentment Over-reliance on people Restricted lifestyle

Coping strategy	Intended consequence	Possible unintended consequences or drawbacks
Drink/drugs (prescribed, over the counter or illegal/ recreational)	Increase feelings of self-confidence Decrease anxiety Increase mood Give a buzz Provide a sense of well-being _____ _____ _____	Out-of-control behaviour and regrets Hangovers/come downs Negative impact on other areas of life Addiction _____ _____ _____
Perfectionism/ Controlling self or others	Avoid criticism Means of controlling anxiety _____ _____ _____	Very hard to achieve and maintain _____ _____ _____
Over-preparation	Increase the likelihood of success Avoid disappointment Decrease anxiety _____ _____ _____	Time-consuming Hard work In certain circumstances increases likelihood of things being stilted and difficult Exhaustion _____ _____ _____

Coping strategy	Intended consequence	Possible unintended consequences or drawbacks
Internally and externally monitoring situations as they happen[14]	Helps you respond quickly to a situation Prevents negative things happening	Hypervigilance can put you on edge Increased likelihood of you noticing negative things Stops you being in and enjoying the moment Attention of others may be drawn to you due to constant checking or appearance of being anxious _____ _____ _____
Pre-mortems and post-mortems (over-thinking a situation before it happens and/or going through it excessively after it has happened)	Prepare yourself for situations Prepare yourself for the possible consequences of situations _____ _____ _____	Increased focus on threat and subsequent anxiety Increased likelihood of predicting or finding problems _____ _____

---

[14] Internal monitoring may mean you are constantly checking your heartrate, your breathing or the thoughts and images in your mind. External monitoring may involve constantly checking others to see if they are looking at you.

Coping strategy	Intended consequence	Possible unintended consequences or drawbacks
Over-planning situations i.e. making sure where the toilet is, where the exit is	Provides quick escape route in the event of difficulties Decrease anxiety	Increases hypervigilance and anxiety in the long run
Self-criticism	Criticize self before someone else does Keep yourself in check Prepares yourself for difficult things that may happen	Lowering of mood Increasing anxiety in the long run
Food fads and constant monitoring of food intake	Avoid rejection on the grounds of how you look While focused on it one can avoid dealing with other things Feeling sense of pride	Eating problems such as bulimia and anorexia
Overeating	Sense of contentment or soothing while eating	Guilt Shame Weight gain & the development of a negative body image

Worksheet 3 : Intended and unintended consequences of your coping strategies

Coping strategy	Intended consequence	Possible unintended consequences or drawbacks
Hurting oneself by cutting/ burning	Sense of release Punishment Controlling emotions	Injury Scars Shame
Wearing make-up excessively	Cover up perceived deficits	Difficult to maintain May warn others off
Constantly apologizing for things	Appease others Decreasing the likelihood that others will attack or reject you	Resentment of others Others may take advantage of you
Seeking reassurance from others	Reduce anxiety	May increase anxiety in the long run as we become reliant on others Others may become frustrated with you and this may affect your relationships

Putting All the Elements Together: Formulation

The following case study is designed to illustrate how all of this information can be drawn together by means of a *formulation*. As with the other case studies in this book, Andy is not a real person but an amalgamation of the stories of several people, in order to protect their confidentiality. Initially a description of key elements in his life will be provided, followed by a formulation of these. After reading Andy's story Exercise 8 will help you develop a formulation based on your own experiences.

Andy's story

Andy was the youngest of three children. He was born with a congenital heart defect, which meant that he had to have surgery when he was very young and regular check-ups until his early twenties. His parents were understandably concerned about his physical well-being and over-protective of him.

At their insistence Andy did not take part in sports at primary school, 'just to be on the safe side', although he wished he could and felt left out and 'different' as a consequence. At secondary school he could take part in certain sports but had to sit out of anything that was thought to be too strenuous, such as cross country, football and sprinting. Secretly Andy worried about his physical health from time to time but did not tell his family as he didn't want to worry them or give them more reason to be over-protective.

His elder brother and sister seemed very confident. When he needed to take the money from his piggy bank to the bank, his sister did it for him. While his brother was a keen football player, Andy was always on the sidelines.

At his all-boys school Andy did well academically. Whenever he had homework he was helped by his brother, sister, mum or dad, and his academic results were good enough for him to gain a university place.

It was at university, while mixing with lots of new people from diverse backgrounds, that Andy started to have difficulties. Many of the people on his course, who lived in the same accommodation, enrolled for sports societies. Although five years previously Andy had received the all clear from his doctors to engage in strenuous physical activity, he had had limited opportunities to develop the skills needed for football and rugby. Everyone his own age had always been so much better than him, and he never got any proper experience of playing with them. He chose not to play sports or go training with the younger boys as he feared he would 'lose face' with his peers. It was easier to say he still had physical health problems, both at school and at university.

Andy missed home but felt stupid saying so to his family, his new set of friends and his old ones. On nights out at university everyone else seemed to be talking about their last football or rugby match or about people he did not know, and he felt excluded. In order to cope, Andy developed the habit of having a couple of drinks before he went out, to give himself some courage, as it seemed to help the flow of conversation. The downside ('unintended consequence') was that a couple of hours later he would find that he was more drunk than everyone else. This was the source of lots of leg pulling from his new friends. Andy laughed along with this, even contributed to or initiated the derogatory comments, but secretly he was feeling more and more socially isolated.

Having had limited contact with girls before going to university, other than those in his family, Andy was very anxious around the opposite sex. He clammed up. Rather than risk looking stupid, he simply avoided speaking to girls and made out to his mates at home that he was seeing a girl at uni, and vice versa.

Constantly finding excuses to go home, Andy spent increasing amounts of time there. His sister and brother had moved away but Andy used his time there to do coursework and catch up with mates from school who hadn't gone away to university. The problem was, he didn't really feel as close to them now either. Sometimes he would sit quietly and listen to them; other times he would invent fictitious events, friendships and conquests, in order to impress his peers.

After university, at the suggestion of his mum and dad, Andy went to work for his uncle in his family business. This was great news, the wage was good and there was no need for endless applications for jobs, something his university mates were finding really frustrating. As time went on, however, he realized some of his new colleagues resented his getting the job 'because he was family'. They seemed to think he was spying for his uncle, and therefore excluded him from their conversations. Andy would watch out for them talking about him, would sit on his own in the canteen pretending to read a book or his texts. Very soon he felt isolated once more. His mood was generally low and he avoided a range of anxiety-provoking situations. He felt ashamed about the way he had 'let things get out of control' and how he was dealing with things now, increasingly telling himself to 'Pull yourself together', asking 'What's wrong with you?', and chiding himself: 'You should be grateful for this job, your health and supportive family – you're pathetic'.

This example can be represented in Diagram 3, though it is important to remember that no formulation will ever give a complete account of someone's life and circumstances. However, it should give an idea of how problems developed for Andy and how they were reinforced by subsequent events.

As you will see, the first box has a range of different influences and experiences that span Andy's life to date. Some of the concerns, strategies and unintended consequences appear to be a direct consequence of his life experiences while others seem to be a consequence of things he has done in order to try to deal with certain problems. In addition it could be argued that some of the 'unintended consequences' could themselves be classed as experiences (and therefore be placed in the first box). What is important is having something that makes sense to the individual and seemingly gives a comprehensive account, via the use of arrows, of how problems have developed and how they are maintained. Remember, the following exercise is for you alone and not something that is going to be scrutinized by others.

Diagram 3: Andy's formulation

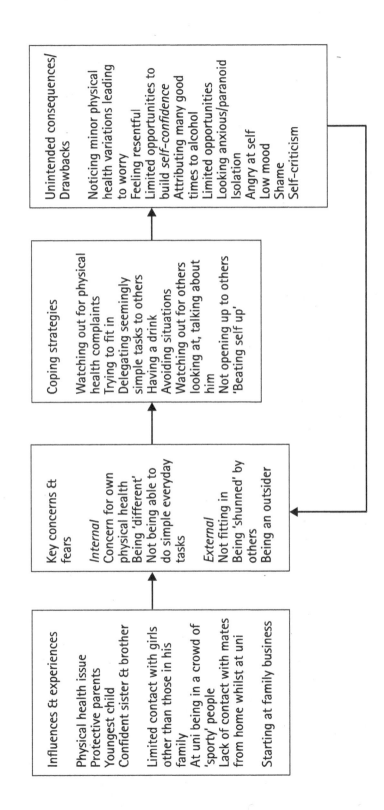

Influences & experiences

Physical health issue
Protective parents
Youngest child
Confident sister & brother

Limited contact with girls other than those in his family
At uni being in a crowd of 'sporty' people
Lack of contact with mates from home whilst at uni

Starting at family business

Key concerns & fears

Internal
Concern for own physical health
Being 'different'
Not being able to do simple everyday tasks

External
Not fitting in
Being 'shunned' by others
Being an outsider

Coping strategies

Watching out for physical health complaints
Trying to fit in
Delegating seemingly simple tasks to others
Having a drink
Avoiding situations
Watching out for others looking at, talking about him
Not opening up to others
'Beating self up'

Unintended consequences/ Drawbacks

Noticing minor physical health variations leading to worry
Feeling resentful
Limited opportunities to build *self-confidence*
Attributing many good times to alcohol
Limited opportunities
Looking anxious/paranoid
Isolation
Angry at self
Low mood
Shame
Self-criticism

Exercise 8: Your own formulation

With the information you have collected in Exercises 6 and 7 now use the blank Diagram 4 (page 63) to develop your own formulation. As you fill in the different boxes it is likely that you will become aware of issues raised in exercises you have previously done that you need to think about more. For example, in Exercise 7 you might have reflected on a way of coping but you may not have noted its potential drawbacks. Or you may have remembered an early life experience in Exercise 6 but not reflected on the key concerns or fears that were associated with it.

If you find it more helpful, use your notebook or journal to draw out the boxes again and fill them in. This may give you more space or help you play around with the content.

When you have completed this exercise, to a point at which you are satisfied you have been able to develop a good account of how your problems developed and how you may inadvertently be maintaining them, it is time to engage in the final exercise of this chapter.

Positive changes in one area can result in positive changes in others

Although this book is aimed at building your self-confidence, it is likely that this exercise will highlight other areas of concern to you, such as anxieties, trauma, low mood and shame. This is because the complexity of human psychology means that it is almost impossible to look at one area of our lives without reflecting on others. Although this may seem complicated, there are also benefits to it. More specifically, working on *one* area can often positively impact on many *other* parts of our psychological lives.

We will come back to this exercise later and review it from a different frame of mind. We will also use it as a focus of compassionate letter writing.

Diagram 4: My own formulation of why problems have developed and how they are maintained

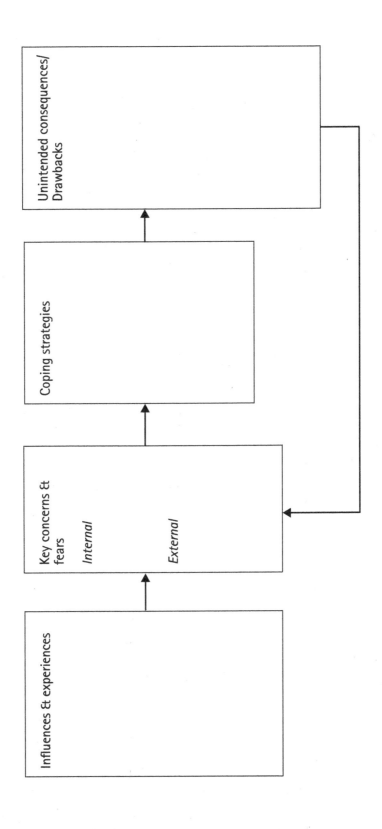

Exercise 9: Making sense of things

Now, standing back from all the emotions generated by the previous exercises in this chapter, look at your formulation as a whole.

Does it make sense of why you are in the situation you find yourself in right now?

If the formulation did not apply to you, but instead to someone you cared about, would it make sense?

If the formulation does not make sense to you, be it in the development of your difficulties or in the way they are maintained, spend a little longer on it.

If you find that you are telling yourself off or undermining yourself in respect of one aspect of the formulation, make a note of it so that you can come back to it later. This may become the focus of imagery work, compassionate letter writing, chair work or compassionate alternative thought worksheets.

Conclusions

We are who we are due to a combination of our biology (nature) and our experiences (nurture). At every point in our life we are attempting to do our best to *get by* or meet our needs, in a difficult world and with a complex brain. Unfortunately, however, the things that we do in order to cope with situations can sometimes have drawbacks in terms of our well-being and self-confidence. Hindsight means that we may all look back on situations and judge ourselves harshly, think that we chose the easier rather than the more helpful option or else simply got things wrong. This may result in self-criticism and self-recrimination.

It is impossible to turn back time and recall all of the reasons why we acted in certain ways at particular points in our life. What is important now is that we attempt to understand ourselves compassionately, learn from experience and nurture both ourselves and our self-confidence.

5 What is Compassion?

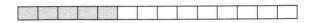

In this chapter we will look at how the *compassionate mind approach* defines compassion. We will examine the compassionate mind or *mindset*[15] in comparison with, and in relation to, different states of mind, such as those we experience in the context of threatening or competitive situations.

We will then discuss the attributes and skills of the compassionate mind (or *mindset*). A better understanding of this will give you an idea of what you are hoping to achieve and also of the skills needed in order to boost your self-confidence.

Traditional Views of Compassion

The majority, if not all, of the early writings on compassion were conducted in the context of religious traditions. Compassion is referred to as a key part of, if not central to, religions such as Jainism, Islam, Buddhism, Judaism, Christianity and Hinduism.

Compassion is viewed slightly differently between the major religions, and even between different texts in the same tradition, but is almost universally accepted to mean, in everyday terms, a deep sympathy and sorrow in the face of suffering, be it our own or that of someone else, *together with* a motivation or commitment to alleviate distress.

Although the compassionate mind approach acknowledges both lay and religious views, it also incorporates or updates our understanding with

---

[15] Within the compassionate mind approach we refer to 'mindsets', which integrate different components or capabilities of our minds, making up a 'set'.

findings from present-day research, which inform us how our brain *orientates* or organizes itself and operates within the context of compassion.

The way in which mindsets work

The following parallel may be a helpful illustration.

You may have experience of applications or 'apps' that turn your phone into a camera, a calculator, a gaming system or an internet connection. In such modes your phone is still a phone but, with different applications running, the keys or areas of the screen behave differently. In turn, you behave differently with the phone, maybe holding it in a different way and viewing it from another angle.

A mindset could be thought of as an 'application' or 'app' for your 'smart brain'. In one mode you can be competitive, resulting in different ways of thinking, different motivations and even different postures. By contrast, engaging with a compassionate mindset will switch the competitive functions off and replace them with a range of different thoughts, motivations and feelings.

Understanding Compassion from the Compassionate Mind Approach

Research suggests that our brains possess a range of mindsets that work in the following ways:

- They orientate our thinking and reasoning (this includes both verbal thoughts and images)

- They orientate our attention

- They recruit certain feelings

- They motivate us towards certain things, resulting in particular behaviours

Different mindsets *turn on* certain functions and capabilities in the brain while *turning off* others. Understanding that compassion is one of these mindsets is a key part of this chapter.

Compassion in contrast to other mindsets

To help us understand mindsets further it may be beneficial briefly to experience and compare different ones in the following three exercises.

Exercise 10: The threat mindset

Imagine, for a moment, you are in a roomful of people and you suddenly notice someone scrutinizing you. Their eyes are narrow and their facial expression suggests they are viewing you in a negative way. This is likely to trigger your *threat* mindset.

After thinking yourself into this mindset, spend a few minutes thoroughly exploring it by answering the questions below:

What is your attention focused on?

What are you thinking?

What emotions do you feel?

What sensations do you feel in your body?

Now let's think about what is likely to have been going on. Your attention will have been narrowed and focused on the threat, and also on yourself in relation to it. It is likely that your thoughts will be fixed on what you think the apparently hostile person is thinking of you. You may start to wonder what is wrong with you, or you may tell yourself they have noticed something you already feel uncomfortable about, maybe with respect to your appearance, your behaviour or you as a person. You may experience anxiety or maybe anger, and these feelings may be associated with a range of different physiological reactions, such as increased heart rate, changes in your breathing pattern and degree of bodily tension. In addition, you may feel motivated to leave, to constantly check if the person is still looking, or to confront the person scrutinizing you.

Finally, take a few deep breaths and let the experience fade from your mind.

Exercise 11: The competitive mindset

Now, imagine you are running a marathon for which you have trained for months and months. You are approaching the final 1000 yards and it looks as though there is a possibility of beating your personal best or even finishing before the rest of your training team. This situation is likely to trigger your *competitive* mindset. After thinking yourself into this mindset, spend a few minutes thoroughly exploring it by answering the questions below.

What is your attention focused on?

What are you thinking?

What emotions do you feel?

What bodily sensations do you feel?

Now let's think about what is likely to have happened. You were probably thinking 'come on', 'push yourself', 'beat your personal best'. Your mind would be full of images of crossing the line, to the cheers of the spectators. If you were thinking about your fellow competitors at all it is unlikely that you were wondering how they were doing. Instead you would have been wondering if you could beat them, or your attention might have been fixed solely on yourself and getting to the finishing line. As you approached it you might have experienced a surge of exhilaration that helped you forget the blisters on your feet and the pain in your limbs. Suddenly you seemed to have a kick of extra energy. You were motivated towards the finishing line and that was all that mattered to you.

Finally, take a few deep breaths and let the experience fade from your mind.

Exercise 12: The compassionate mindset

Imagine for a moment that you are visiting a friend or colleague for the first time since they suffered a bereavement. On the way you may initially wonder how the visit will go, whether you will be of any help to them, and maybe feel a bit anxious about it. As they open the door you notice a look of profound sorrow on their face, tears in their eyes. This situation is likely to trigger your *compassionate* mindset. After thinking yourself into this mindset, spend a few minutes thoroughly exploring it by answering the questions below.

What is your attention focused on?

What are you thinking?

What emotions do you feel?

What bodily sensations do you feel?

Now let's think about what is likely to have happened. As soon as you encounter the bereaved person, your thoughts will be directed towards them and how they are feeling. Any thoughts of yourself and your own concerns about the visit will be set aside. You may feel physically drawn towards the other person, or the need to make eye contact. You may experience a deep sense of sorrow, and the need to be of help to them (in whatever way they seem to require at that moment). This may mean giving them a hug, talking or 'taking them out of themselves' by going for a drink with them and filling them in on what has been happening.

Once again, take a few deep breaths and let the experience fade from your mind.

Reflections on Exercises 10 to 12

As you can see from the scenarios described above, we all have the capacity for different mindsets that organize our brains in different ways. Some make us focus on ourselves, some on other people; some drive us towards certain things, some away from them.

In each of the scenarios outlined we are still 'ourselves' but the ways in which our brains operate are different.

So what have mindsets got to do with developing self-confidence?

This book aims to help you develop self-confidence through a compassionate mindset. In Chapter 1 we saw that although warmth and kindness are central to compassion, so too are strength and courage. A compassionate mindset will help you recognize when things are difficult, and have the strength and courage to do something about it instead of constantly undermining yourself and your efforts.

Exercise 13: Comparing different mindsets

The following exercise will illustrate further how different mindsets compare with each other, and how the development of your compassionate mindset may stand you in good stead.

Let's return to Jim and Becky's story from the first chapter. As you will recall, Jim wanted to ask Becky out, but when he bumped into her his self-confidence failed him. He ended up talking about something completely different. He found himself in a threat mindset. Thinking about this situation, jot down some ideas in the middle column ('Threat mindset') of worksheet 4 provided overleaf. Think about what thoughts Jim might have had, where his attention might have been, how he might have been feeling and what he was motivated to do. It is important to remember that the exercise is asking you to think about what might have been happening for Jim while he was 'in' the situation – not before or after but when he actually bumped into Becky.

Now, in contrast, imagine that in the crucial moment Jim was able to be compassionate towards himself. In this mindset he still experiences anxiety, and is not impervious to life's setbacks and disappointments, but he feels reassured that he will be OK whatever situations face him and that he can recover from any knocks he takes. He is able to keep his anxiety in check so that his threat system is not allowed to 'run the show'. Now with this mindset, complete the second column of the worksheet ('Compassionate mindset').

As you can see from each of the exercises in this chapter, different mindsets can influence our thinking, attention, bodily sensations, motivation, behaviour and even our posture, in startlingly different ways. The aim is not to rid yourself of anxiety altogether but rather to be able to keep it in check by developing a compassionate mindset for your situation, through which you can learn to regulate your threat system and build your self-confidence.

Worksheet 4 : Threat mindset versus compassionate mindset

	Threat mindset	Compassionate mindset
What thoughts might have been running through Jim's mind?		
Where would Jim's attention be focused?		
What emotions is Jim likely to experience?		
What feelings might Jim experience in his body?		
How might Jim hold himself/what would his posture be likely to be in this situation?		
What would Jim be motivated to do?		

You may have found the last exercise difficult as we have yet to look specifically at the different components of compassion and the associated qualities. If this was the case for you it may be helpful to return to the exercise after reading the rest of this chapter.

How do mindsets and their associated emotions relate to each other?

As mentioned previously, our mindsets are each associated with a particular way of thinking, feeling, different motivations and behaviours. Thus they recruit or switch on certain functions of the brain. Although mindsets can sometimes be associated with a mixture of different emotions, there are certain emotions that do not have the capacity to co-exist with others. In other words, one negates the other. This occurs naturally, but human beings are also able to manipulate it to their advantage. For example, research has demonstrated that if an individual is induced into a state of relaxation, they cannot simultaneously feel anxious; one state counteracts the other. It is through the intervention of the compassionate mind or mindset that you will hopefully become able to turn down or turn off the sometimes troublesome threat system.

Looking Further at the Compassionate Mind or Mindset: Compassionate Attributes

After decades of research Paul Gilbert has distinguished six *attributes* (or qualities) of compassion that are all experienced in the context of emotional warmth. Warmth is important as it turns something that could be a purely intellectual concept into something with much greater emotional resonance. The attributes are distinct but they are also very closely related and complement each other. Each one is outlined below together with a brief indication of how it may apply to your own efforts to build your self-confidence.

Care for well-being

This attribute involves a commitment and motivation to truly care for the well-being of yourself and/or others.

Care for well-being may mean making a commitment to face something we feel anxious about because we *know* it is in our best interests to *do* so, even if it is something we are fearful of doing.

Sensitivity to distress

This involves noticing when you, or others, are distressed and/or experiencing difficult emotions. It also involves being open to such things in order that you notice them.

The fact that you are reading this book suggests that you have noticed you are experiencing some difficulty with self-confidence. However, it is important that this sensitivity is coupled with warmth in order that hostile thoughts, such as 'I've got to pull myself together/sort myself out', turn into nurturing ones, such as 'I'm having a difficult time and it would be helpful if I acknowledged this and took steps to help myself.'

Sympathy

This is the ability to be moved by our situation, or that of others, and connect with the pain experienced.

Sympathy in relation to difficulties with your self-confidence may involve recognizing (with warmth): 'This is hard, and it's understandable that I struggle in this way.'

Empathy

Empathy allows us to think about the nature of our minds and those of others. It allows us to see things from different perspectives and, in the context of our difficulties, think about what we, or someone else, may need.

In relation to our self-confidence, empathy may help us work out exactly what we need at that specific point in time. This, of course, is very similar to 'care for well-being'.

Non-judgement

This involves understanding that human beings are complex. It is about being non-condemnatory of things that occur in our lives and in our minds, or those of others. This is in contrast to being judgemental, which is often associated with shame and criticism of ourselves and/ or others. Non-judgement does not, however, mean being detached. Remember, all of these attributes are experienced within the context of warmth.

Hopefully, after reading the material outlined in Chapters 1 to 3 and 'making sense of your experiences' in Chapter 4, you will now be able to view yourself as a human being who, like many others, struggles with certain things. Viewing yourself in this way helps reduce self-criticism and shame, while also increasing a non-judgemental warmth in relation to the things that have happened to you and the situation you find yourself in right now.

Distress tolerance

This attribute involves feeling difficult emotions despite an urge to suppress them or push them away. Such emotions may include anxiety, sadness, anger, jealousy or guilt. Although at times it may be important to keep our emotions in check, it is imperative that we do not do this all the time as this is widely considered to lie at the root of many psychological difficulties.

In relation to our self-confidence, being able to tolerate distress involves acknowledging the emotions we feel and giving them space. It may involve resisting the urge to avoid a problem and lead you to 'feel the fear and do it anyway'.[16]

Skills of the Compassionate Mind or Mindset

In addition to compassionate attributes, this approach also distinguishes a number of *skills* (or things that we can learn to *do*) to help harness and maintain the compassionate mind or mindset. Similar to the compassionate attributes, these skills are very closely related to each other and are outlined below:

Compassionate understanding

This practice involves understanding the reasons why we are as we are and the situations we subsequently find ourselves in. It involves being supportive of ourselves and others.

Compassionate imagery

When we are anxious it is very easy to generate frightening images in our minds, images from the past or from the predicted future. Maybe in the moment we experience self-critical ones. Compassionate images are supportive, understanding, kind and encouraging, and can be used to help us.

Compassionate attention

This allows us to recognize when things went well, or maybe times when they didn't but things turned out OK anyway, and to learn from this in contrast to always focusing on the negative. It also helps us focus on things in a way that helps balance any negatives we may perceive or experience.

---

[16] The title of a book by Susan Jeffers.

Compassionate motives

These direct you towards things that enable you to flourish in the long term, supporting your well-being. Compassionate motives can also be experienced in relation to others.

Compassionate behaviour

Such actions emerge from compassionate motives and involve us acting in a way that is beneficial for our own well-being or that of others.

Compassionate emotions

Feelings of warmth, support, kindness and a sense of connectedness.

How Do These Attributes and Skills Fit Together?

Imagine a six-legged stool (see Diagram 5, page 78). Each leg would represent one of the six attributes of compassion. Such a frame would provide a solid and strong base. Remove any of the legs and the stool would still be stable – but a little less so. Now imagine that the stool seat is made up of a tight six-way cane weave, each strand representing one of the compassionate skills.

These attributes and skills are integral to building and maintaining compassion. The more compassionate attributes and skills you can develop and use, the more robust your compassionate mind will be. But of course if you struggle with certain attributes, don't worry as the structure still has a considerable amount of strength. Proceed with what you can do and maybe return to the things you find difficult later on. The structure of the stool represents compassion, the platform upon which you will build self-confidence.

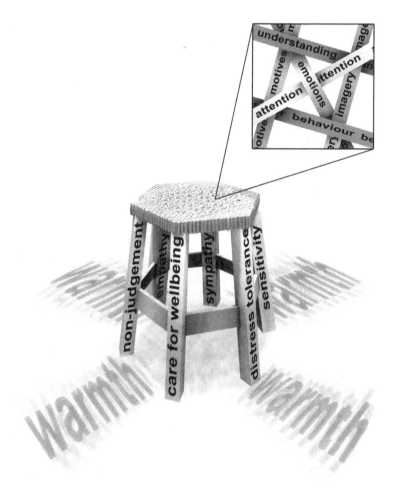

Diagram 5: The compassion stool

How Do We Gain Such Attributes and Skills?

It is likely that although you may have these attributes and skills in relation to others, you may not often use them on yourself. This is, of course, very common. As the skills and attributes outlined are central to cornerstones of developing self-compassion, and ultimately building your self-confidence, they will become the focus of later chapters in this book.

Conclusions

So far we have learnt that compassion is a *mindset*. When we engage with our compassionate mind, we turn off certain capacities and abilities in the brain while turning on others. The same can be said for threat or competitive mindsets. Six compassionate attributes and six skills form the firm foundation on which self-confidence is built.

6 Obstacles to the Development of Self-compassion

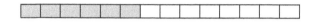

Although many people have no problem with being compassionate *to* others, accepting compassion *from* others and practising *self*-compassion can be a different matter for them. This can ultimately interfere with their ability to build self-confidence.

The biggest obstacles that can prevent us from accepting compassion from others, and exercising self-compassion, are the *views and thoughts* we may hold about compassion and about ourselves.

Emotional and environmental obstacles can also be very powerful indeed, and can catch us unawares. For example, feelings of self-compassion may bring up difficult and seemingly surprising emotions and memories that can interfere with the work involved in building self-confidence. Others find that people close to them resist the changes they attempt to make, maybe because they have got used to seeing them in a certain way.

This chapter will look at some of the obstacles to self-compassion, and their potential origins. It will focus on why such obstacles also impact on the development of self-confidence. We will then think about the ways in which you can negotiate these.

Common Obstacles to Accepting Compassion from Others and/or Self-compassion

Whether you are aware of some level of personal resistance to developing self-compassion or not, it may be helpful to you to read through the statements below and mark those that resonate with you.

Ten Views and Thoughts that can be Obstacles to Self-compassion

1.   Self-compassion is about self-pity   ☐

Pity *for others* is often viewed as synonymous with 'looking down' from a position of superiority or feeling 'sorry for' someone, while pity *for the self* is often dismissed as wallowing. For many, pity means that an individual's innate strength and resilience is not acknowledged; they are defined solely by the situation they find themselves in rather than as a whole person. If this is how you define pity then self-compassion is absolutely not about 'self-pity'.

It is, however, important to recognize that different people and cultures view the concept of pity in different ways. Literal translations have resulted in further confusion surrounding the concept. For example, Michelangelo's '*Pietà*' is a Christian work of art depicting the mother of Christ holding her dead son's body. When many Italians speak of the sculpture they reflect that, for them, this is the depiction of ultimate love and compassion. Within their culture '*pietà*' is not a negative thing at all.

2.   Self-compassion is about being selfish or self-centred   ☐

In fact, self-compassion often brings with it a greater capacity to help oneself *and,* in turn, others. Having become more self-compassionate, people often report having greater strength to deal with conflicts and become better friends, parents and colleagues.

Lack of self-compassion by contrast means that we are more likely to become immobilized or consumed by our own difficulties and therefore less able to help others.

3.   I don't deserve compassion   ☐

Self-compassion can be blocked by the belief that we are not worthy or deserving of it. If you feel you don't deserve compassion it is likely that you are judging yourself or your actions negatively and experiencing high levels of shame. As we saw in Chapter 3 this can undermine the development of your self-confidence.

If you identify with this, hopefully the work you did in Chapter 4, which involved developing an understanding of your journey and the situation you find yourself in now, will have gone some way to addressing this. Later we will use compassionate imagery to help you review your formulation from Chapter 4. A sense of 'not deserving' can also be used as the focus of compassionate alternative thought worksheets and compassionate letter writing later on.

For now, however, it may be helpful to think of your own sense of 'non-deserving' as a fear that is challenging but not overwhelming. Encourage yourself to take things one small step at a time. Ask yourself, 'What aspect of compassion don't I deserve?' and start with the ones that you feel you do. Start slowly. As you work on specific areas, you may find that self-compassion may be a good thing, without the drawbacks you predicted. In other words, you won't suddenly become a bad person, get found out by others and be humiliated if you practise them. And once the ball is rolling you may find that you actually want to try on for size other aspects of self-compassion.

If feeling 'non-deserving' really is tripping you up, there are two further things you could try. First, it may be of benefit to get someone else's opinion as to whether or not you deserve compassion. This may be someone you trust such as a family member or friend. Alternatively it may be of help to you to seek professional advice by asking for a referral to a therapist.

4. **My needs are not as important as other people's**   ☐

For some, personal needs (including the need for self-compassion) are put on the back burner in favour of the needs of others. This is a classic trap many people fall into. But when we perpetually put the needs of others first we can subsequently feel a sense of anger and resentment. We feel taken for granted; we may feel as though we are not cared for, and become exhausted. Although we all do this at times, it is important that this way of thinking does not become extreme and immobilizing. Compassion is about striking a balance between focusing on ourselves and on others.

Even if you still think that the needs of others are more important than yours, start practising self-compassion *because* you are doing it for them. You can always revert back to your old ways if you find it doesn't help.

5. **Self-compassion is about letting yourself off the hook**   ❑

Key to self-compassion is understanding the things that *have* happened and the things we *have* done, as well as the things that *are* happening and which we *are* doing. With a more balanced perspective on them, hopefully we can move away from self-criticism and shame. However, being understanding of yourself does not mean relinquishing responsibility, excusing your own actions or letting yourself off the hook. Where appropriate, self-compassion is about taking responsibility for the things we might have done or continue to do. It then involves committing ourselves, wherever possible, to changing things for the better. This will hopefully be beneficial both to ourselves and others, as is illustrated by Tom's story.

Tom's story

Tom had found himself being sarcastic towards others and keeping them at arm's length. People had commented that he could be 'difficult' and some members of his family were no longer in contact with him. Through Tom's work on developing self-compassion he finally began to face his own role in the development and maintenance of his current difficulties, something he had always previously resisted. Instead of being self-critical about it, he began to understand why he had acted in certain ways. It was understandable given some of the difficulties he had faced. With a compassionate mindset he was able to resolve conflicts, adjust his behaviour and repair his relationships – or, as he put it, he began to face up to things.

Of course sometimes we 'put ourselves on the hook' because we feel we deserve it. This clearly overlaps with the feeling of non-deserving outlined before. If this applies to you it may be of help to ask your-self: 'What elements of compassion do I deserve?' and start from there.

6. **Self-compassion is a weak or a soft option** ☐

Contrary to what many people believe, developing self-compassion is *not* the weak or soft option. It involves facing our difficulties and experiencing a range of emotions that are uncomfortable. It then requires the motivation or commitment to change ourselves, which requires courage and strength.

In the context of building your self-confidence, compassion may involve speaking up for yourself despite an overwhelming urge not to. It may involve facing your fears and doing something while every part of your being may seem to be arguing against it. It may involve letting people see the 'true you' and letting down your guard. All of this takes strength and courage.

7. **Compassion lets your guard down and leaves you open to threat** ☐

Thanks to our brain's 'better safe than sorry' default setting and per-haps some adverse life experiences, our threat system often ends up 'running the show'. This isn't very efficient and, bottom line, it's not very comfortable to be on edge much of the time either.

Practising self-compassion can actually make your threat system run more efficiently; it makes you wiser and helps you decide when you need to put your guard up and when you don't. For example, if you live in a hostile environment self-compassion will help you protect yourself. However, in relatively safe environments it will give you the strength to face difficult situations and build your self-confidence.

If you find this is a particular obstacle for you I would recommend that you keep your guard up as much as you want. But, as time goes on, by practising self-compassion you may find that you are better

able to distinguish when you need to protect yourself and when protection may be a waste of effort.

8. **Allowing myself to experience positive feelings will
    set me up for a fall** ❑

Sometimes people are wary of positive moods or feelings of calmness or relaxation. Such experiences are associated with a fear that
they are setting themselves up for a fall or that something may come
out of the blue that they weren't prepared for. Alternatively some
believe that feeling good will attract negative things – or payback.
This is illustrated by Peter's story below.

Peter's story

Peter had suffered a number of setbacks in his life, such as being
made redundant and his first girlfriend splitting up from him. These
events seemed to arrive out of the blue, so he started to be wary of
such things happening again. Of course it was difficult for Peter ever
to know whether being watchful would have prevented the redundancy or the break-up. But it was certainly true that his strategy of
constantly watching over his shoulder was now interfering with his
life and wasn't doing him any good. His hypervigilance had even
been cited by a subsequent girlfriend as the reason why she broke off
their relationship. On balance he wished he could return to the old
carefree days.

Self-compassion can actually be the best way of preparing yourself for
the difficulties and setbacks that life inevitably brings. This is because
it builds your ability to cope with such situations. It is through setbacks
that self-confidence in our ability to cope with life's knocks is increased.
If this obstacle applies to you it may be helpful just to think, 'I'll give it a
go. I can always revert to my old ways.'

Obviously this section of the book is focusing on *views and thoughts* that
may form obstacles to acquiring self-compassion. Later in this chapter

we will reflect on how certain emotions can become paired with each other in the brain. This can lead to the experience of difficult emotions swiftly succeeding pleasurable ones.

9. **Self-compassion means not facing up to difficult emotions**   ☐

This is one of the most common misunderstandings relating to self-compassion. In fact, it is about facing up to and experiencing difficult emotions rather than turning away from them. Such emotions include sadness, anxiety and anger. It's about *owning and validating* such emotions, and allowing ourselves to work through them instead of bottling them up, with adverse consequences for our mental well-being.

Self-compassion can help you develop the strength and courage to put yourself in anxiety-provoking situations in order to build your self-confidence. If you wait till you feel confident enough to do something, you may be waiting a long time. Often we need to act first in order to start to feel self-confidence.

10. **It will be too hard or too overwhelming**   ☐

For some, the thought of experiencing compassion, from others or from themselves, can evoke fear. Emotions that have been bottled up may come bursting out, with a destabilizing effect. Although learning to practise self-compassion can be difficult, as mentioned previously, suppression of emotions is thought to underpin many psychological difficulties. Working on them with self-compassion instead, though difficult in the short term, can ultimately be extremely rewarding.

Here are some strategies that can help:

• Go at a pace that is comfortable for you.

• Start gradually. Remember, if you were learning to swim you would begin by buying a swimsuit or trunks, find out about pool opening hours and begin at the shallow end. Approach your work with self-compassion in a similar way.

- Engage in the work at a time when you feel you have the resources and/or support to do it.

- Do the work alongside the introduction of pleasurable activities, such as increasing contact with good friends, planning some time for yourself, going for walks or engaging in other forms of exercise.

- Time it for when your life is relatively stable and stress-free.

- If you feel that you need the support of a professional, speak to your GP about getting some form of psychological therapy.

Emotional Obstacles to Experiencing Self-compassion

Sometimes while attempting to build our self-confidence people are surprised to find difficult emotions and associated memories surfacing in their mind. This can seem extremely confusing. Elaine's story may help illustrate this.

Elaine's story

Elaine had found the mindfulness components of our therapeutic work together really helpful, but felt overwhelming anxiety and tinges of anger when we moved on to engaging with exercises aimed at evoking self-compassion. She had experienced similar emotions when she disclosed difficult things during the early days of therapy, but had explained it away to herself as a consequence of the process of getting to know her therapist. Although this was partially true, it was also an early indicator of the emotions she was to experience later.

Together we reviewed Elaine's early-life experiences in order to make sense of these emotions, and she disclosed that her parents had been very unpredictable in their responses to her at key times in her life. Sometimes they were comforting, but other times dismissive or even punishing. Elaine recalled a number of significant memories. For example, one day she had fallen from her bike and run screaming to her step-mum. Instead of the comfort she had sought, her screams were met with anger. Although Elaine said that she thought she had 'dealt with these things' previously, such events made sense of why self-compassion evoked difficult emotions for her in the present. Understanding this was a key element to our work together. Noticing and accepting such emotions, talking and allowing herself to feel them, were pivotal to her becoming more self-compassionate.

The psychological concept of 'conditioning' as well as neuroscience research accounts for why some individuals have emotions that seemingly become paired with others. I find that the phrase 'neurons that fire together wire together' encapsulates this very simply. In basic terms, if we are punished for feeling anger as a child, it is likely that anger will become paired with anxiety (the anxiety we feel before, during or after the punishment) in adult life. Anger may occur simultaneously with anxiety or seemingly be replaced by it (in other words, situations that are likely to produce anger produce anxiety instead). In a second example, if a child goes to their parent when they are upset and, instead of receiving a hug, they are repeatedly ignored, rejected or even humiliated, that child will begin to link the experience of needing closeness with the experience of anger, anxiety or sadness. While they are young they may learn not to approach their parent, but as an adult they may experience confusing emotions whenever they feel a sense of closeness to someone.

These strong and seemingly contradictory emotions can also be paired with vivid memories. Sometimes the emotion comes first, sometimes the memory, and at other times we experience them simultaneously. Although some individuals find that such memories are useful to them as they help account for why they are feeling certain emotions, other people find them extremely difficult to handle. Deborah Lee has written *A Compassionate Mind Approach to Recovering From Trauma*, which focuses on emotional memories relating to traumatic experiences. If you feel this describes your situation, her book may be helpful to you.

So emotions can become linked or 'wired' together. They can also be paired with difficult memories that burst into our minds uninvited. The feeling of compassion may subsequently evoke fear, anxiety, sadness and anger. Understanding this can be the first step to dealing with it. We can then endeavour to work through the emotions and hopefully use compassion to soothe the difficult feelings.

Of course, if you find that this is too difficult to do on your own then there is no shame in seeking the help and advice of others. Your GP may be a good starting point to direct you to further help.

Environmental Obstacles to Building Self-confidence

Many people who are attempting to build their own self-compassion and self-confidence find others around them resisting the significant changes they are attempting to make. Have a look at the following three stories.

Henry's story

Henry developed the strength and motivation to start putting himself forward for things at work – things he would never have dreamt of attempting in the past. When he first volunteered himself to chair a future meeting, everyone in his department turned round and looked at him in shock. Two people even sniggered while another stated, in a patronizing tone, 'Are you sure?' This made Henry more anxious than ever. At the meeting, the following week, more people than usual turned up. At difficult points he noticed people rolling their eyes, or once again sniggering, as if they were just watching and waiting for him to mess up. He found people talked over him, in a way they didn't seem to do with more confident members of the team, and they were more likely to carry on conversations when he asked for certain discussions to come to an end.

Emma's story

Emma found that her sister and brother seemed to block her attempts to build her self-confidence. When she eventually plucked up the courage to put a point across to them about the care of their parents, they seemed to ignore what she was saying, quickly returning to their own discussion. In the past Emma had always reluctantly gone along with their suggestions, fearful of how they would respond to her putting a different opinion forward. Now, as she attempted to make her point, she was continually overruled by them. It was almost as if she had to 'over-assert' herself if she was going to get anywhere, because simply putting her own point of view was getting her nowhere.

Patricia's story

After never saying yes to nights out with work colleagues, Patricia decided that this was something she would like to change. Just getting an invitation, however, proved to be difficult. Eventually she had to invite herself. When making plans for getting to and from the venue, she found that everyone else had already arranged shared taxis and lifts, based on previous nights out. She lived the farthest away and in consequence had to plan to leave early so as to get the last train home. All in all, it felt as though she wasn't really welcome and was viewed as an inconvenience by everybody else even before the night started.

The situations in which Henry, Emma and Patricia found themselves were extremely difficult. It was almost as if they had to work even harder than everyone else just to receive an appropriate response, respect or inclusion.

If you identify with the stories above, the exercises in Chapter 12 may be used to problem-solve around such situations, breaking things down into manageable steps.

Of course, at times being more self-compassionate means thinking about whether we really need to change our environment. Do we want certain people in our lives any longer, such as those who make us feel bad and do not change the way they behave around us, despite our best efforts to alter the situation? Self-compassion can help us with this as it gives us the courage to face up to things but also, when necessary, to walk away from them.

What Has This Got to Do with Developing Self-confidence?

In Chapter 3 we suggested that most people would want the compassionate teacher for their child, rather than the disciplinarian: a teacher who nurtures their development, looks at difficulties and mistakes as opportunities to learn and grow, and is open and warm. It is interesting that intuitively we know what will help others, but in contrast often find that our own 'inner teacher' is hostile and critical – a carping voice that tells us that we are stupid, pathetic, a waste of space, and unable to do certain things in certain areas of our life. This can result in us simply 'shutting down', avoiding situations or 'putting a face on'. But if we can learn to adopt a more self-compassionate approach to our difficulties, we can build our self-confidence step by step. We can nurture ourselves into a state of well-being which provides us with the resilience we need to take life's knocks as they come and then move forward again.

If you have identified with any of the obstacles outlined in this chapter it may be helpful to you to read the following section. If, on the other hand, you do not perceive any potential blocks to self-compassion you may decide to move on to the next chapter.

Ideas for negotiating the obstacles to self-compassion

In the process of reading this chapter you may have started to realize that self-compassion is not about letting yourself off the hook, venting emotions and setting yourself up for a fall. Instead, adopting a self-compassionate mindset involves employing strength and courage to face difficult things, as well as tolerating and being sensitive to your own distress and that of others. In the following exercise you will be provided with a further means by which you may objectively negotiate obstacles. Let's look again at Patricia's story. She identified two main obstacles that were holding her back.

1. Accepting compassion from others

I feared this would leave me open to upset and disappointment later. It is easier to disregard compassion from others, preferring to think that 'people are only saying that' and 'if they really knew me they wouldn't feel that way'.

2. Developing self-compassion

This would ultimately mean dropping my guard and would result in me not being prepared for things that happened in the future.

Despite these concerns Patricia was also worried that if she did not do anything, she would continue to be 'walked all over' by others and never be able to achieve the things she wanted to achieve within her work and personal life.

Having initially identified her personal obstacles, Patricia then looked at the pros and cons of both accepting compassion from others and developing self-compassion. This was done by completing the worksheets below.

Patricia's worksheet: Listing the pros and cons of accepting compassion from others and developing self-compassion

Cons of accepting compassion from others	Pros of accepting compassion from others
I may be disappointed by people later I won't be as ready for being let down	It may be a nice thing to do It may help me challenge some of my own undermining It may mean that I begin to feel more self-confident if I feel the support of others around me I may get a 'warm glow'
Cons of developing self-compassion	**Pros of developing self-compassion**
I may drop my guard and be less able to spot problems	Life may be easier I may not be walked over as much as I may feel stronger It may help me achieve what I want to achieve because life may be less stressful It may stop me undermining myself It may develop my self-confidence

On balance it seemed as though working on developing Patricia's self-compassionate mind, as a means of building her self-confidence, might be worthwhile.

Following on from this she looked at each of the potential obstacles associated with both accepting compassion from others and developing self-compassion, by means of problem-solving around such concerns. Patricia's completed problem-solving worksheet can be found on page 74.

Patricia's worksheet: Completed problem-solving worksheet

Things to tell myself and things I can do to address my concerns
If I become disappointed later I can use self-compassion to help me with this.
If I am let down I can remind myself that I have been let down before and come through it – this time will hopefully be different, though, as I am addressing the habit of self-criticism. I may also be able to go to other people, who haven't let me down, for their support.
I have learnt that compassion isn't about dropping your guard but helping it work more efficiently. I am not leaving myself unprotected.
I can always revert to my old ways if I need to do so.

This closer examination of compassion and self-compassion ultimately resulted in Patricia deciding to 'give it a go'. Although still a little sceptical, she decided it might be useful to try something new, if only so that she could say she had done so.

Exploring the Obstacles You May Need to Negotiate

Exercise 14: My obstacles to experiencing compassion from others

Using the categories you have ticked in the 'common obstacles' section of this chapter, or others that you may be aware of, list below any obstacles that you think may restrict or prevent you from experiencing compassion from others.

_____

_____

_____

_____

_____

_____

_____

_____

_____

_____

_____

_____

_____

_____

_____

_____

_____

_____

_____

_____

_____

_____

_____

Exercise 15: My obstacles to developing self-compassion

Once again using the categories you have ticked in the 'common obstacles' section of this chapter, or others that you may be aware of, list below any obstacles that you think may restrict or prevent you from developing self-compassion.

_____

_____

_____

_____

_____

_____

_____

_____

_____

_____

_____

_____

_____

_____

_____

_____

_____

_____

_____

_____

_____

_____

_____

_____

_____

_____

_____

_____

Exercise 16: The pros and cons of accepting compassion from others

Starting initially with the first two columns in worksheet 5, explore the pros and cons you are aware of with respect to accepting compassion from others.

Worksheet 5: Accepting compassion from others

Pros	Cons	Things you can do or say to yourself to help you with these cons

Exercise 17: The pros and cons of developing self-compassion

Similarly, starting initially with the first two columns in worksheet 6, explore the pros and cons of developing self-compassion.

Worksheet 6 : Developing self-compassion

Pros	Cons	Things you can do or say to yourself to help you with these cons

Exercise 18: Problem-solving around your concerns

As you will have noticed, worksheets 5 and 6 are composed of three columns, with the third asking you to make a note of things you can do or say to yourself to help with the cons.

Going back to each worksheet you have completed, spend a little time reflecting on what measures you can take to help you cope with these obstacles. This may involve things that you can say to yourself or things that you can do.

Conclusions

Obstacles to self-compassion are common. They can come in the form of the views and thoughts which we have developed over time in response to our environment, from emotional obstacles, and from pressure from those around us. Some are relatively easy to overcome, others less so. If the ground covered in this chapter helps you move forward towards practising self-compassion this is good news.

There are a number of exercises later in this book that may help you further negotiate the obstacles. And it may be of help to come back to this section again, having read the later part of the book and developed new skills.

7 Preparing for Compassion Using Mindfulness

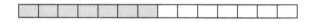

Introducing the Concept of 'Self-practice'

In this section, and throughout the rest of the book, I will be introducing a range of exercises for you to try. Some you will find useful, others perhaps less so. Once you have found exercises to suit you, you will be encouraged to engage in these regularly in what is referred to as 'self-practice'.

In the same way as you may develop a helpful routine at the gym or a system for keeping on top of housework, your 'self-practice' will hopefully be made up of things that you find useful and with which you engage regularly.

You will recall that at the start of the book, on page xxviii, there is a personal practice summary sheet on which to note your ongoing thoughts on the exercises in this book. You can then refer to these notes in the final chapter when you are putting together your personal plan for future self-practice.

For the time being, however, approach these exercises in a spirit of curiosity and 'try them out' as if you were trying new food or a new hobby. The important thing is to remain open-minded and not let preconceptions prevent you from experimenting. Of course I am not suggesting you should continue to do something you don't like or find distasteful, but it is important to give things a go.

Mindfulness

We have seen how evolution provided human beings with the amazing ability to think about the past, present and future. This has been hugely important for our survival. Unfortunately, however, this ability also means that we can find ourselves dwelling on past situations and predicting catastrophes in the future. All of this can activate our threat system and prevent our self-confidence from developing.

So how do we give our minds a break and stop getting caught up in the seemingly never-ending drama that goes on inside our heads? One approach that people are increasingly finding helpful is something that originated in the Eastern religious traditions: mindfulness. More recently, mindfulness has been developed in the west as a practice to promote well-being. The approach has been found to be of help to a wide range of individuals, from those who consider themselves to be psychologically 'well' to those who identify themselves as suffering from anxiety and depression, amongst other difficulties.

The practice of mindfulness involves bringing one's complete attention and calm awareness to the present moment – an awareness containing curiosity and non-judgement. This may involve paying attention to things going on around us or to the thoughts occurring in our mind. The practice aims to help us:

- slow things down

- be in the present moment (instead of everywhere but)

- become more observant about what is going on in our minds

- make and implement choices about what we pay attention to, instead of letting our threat or drive system run the show

- ultimately help us 'feel' better and make better choices about whether or not to act on thoughts and feelings

Within the practice, when we become *mindful* that our attention has wandered from the moment, the key is to notice where our mind has moved to and *without judgement* but with *curiosity* bring the mind and attention back into focus.

Our mind's tendency to wander

Our minds wander all the time and this is perfectly normal. Sometimes they are drawn to sounds, feelings, sensations, thoughts of what we are going to have for tea or what we watched on the TV last night. They will be particularly drawn to things that are 'on your mind'. This may be something we need to do, something that has already been done, something we are looking forward to, or something we need to prepare for. The art of mindfulness means, in that moment when we realize our mind has wandered, gently bringing our attention back to what we wish to focus on. Often I have made a whole list of things to do before I realize I have moved my focus, but when I realize this I gently adjust and bring it back to the practice.

I hope that this new skill will be helpful to you. I also hope it will act as the foundation stone for a whole range of exercises to be introduced later, aimed at helping you build your compassionate mind. In turn we can then use your compassionate mind to build your self-confidence.

Mindfulness can be both difficult and easy

Some people find it difficult because they fall into the trap of striving 'to get it right'; their drive or threat system kicks in and takes over. Others may become panicky when they try these exercises, and if this is the case for you there are some ideas later that may help with this. For all of us, the busyness of our brains and the complexity of our lives mean that there can be inbuilt obstacles to mindfulness practice – that said, this could also be the most compelling reason to adopt it. On the positive side, mindfulness is something that can be easily practised, doesn't need special equipment, and requires only time and motivation. It can be practised while going for a walk, sitting quietly, while in a busy place or even while washing your hands.

I will now take you through a number of different exercises. If you can, try each one a number of times over a period of a week or so, and see also if you can increase the length of time you spend engaging in the exercises.

When I am talking people through these exercises I aim to do so in a relaxed and soothing manner. The tone of my voice is soft and my speech is a lot slower than usual. I have tried to convey this by the way I have written down the exercises, using lots of suspension points to convey pauses and slowing down. As there is no way to convey a tone of voice in writing, I will merely suggest that, as you talk yourself through these exercises (be it out loud or with your inner voice), do so in a tone of gentleness and curiosity.

I hope you will return to and use certain of these exercises later, and for this reason each one is written out in full.

Exercise 19 : Mindfulness of sound

Start by finding a location that is, as far as possible, free from major distractions. This place could be somewhere in your home, in your garden, in a park or any other place you think may be suitable. It is a good idea to make yourself comfortable. This may mean sitting on a chair or bench, on the ground, or maybe on a sofa or bed.

Allow 10–15 minutes for this as you may find the exercise helpful and soothing, and wish to stay with it for some time.

Ideally I would recommend that you sit in an upright posture, with your feet on the floor approximately hip-distance apart, your hands gently resting in your lap. Feel a strength in your spine, yet a relaxation in your body and a sense of openness. If this position is difficult or feels uncomfortable, or if you would just prefer to do the exercise with legs crossed or while lying down, that is OK. The most important thing is to feel comfortable with your body and its position in order that you can immerse yourself in the exercise as fully as possible.

It is helpful if you can close your eyes for this exercise, knowing that at any time you can open them if you wish. Others may prefer to settle their gaze on a fixed point on the floor or somewhere low down.

Begin by noticing the sounds that are around you............maybe the song of a bird............the babble of water............the sound of the wind in the trees............maybe the hum of a computer............cars driving by............the banging of pipes............the rumble of your belly.

Notice them getting louder or quieter............notice them coming and going............notice them with curiosity and without judgement.

When there are no sounds observe the silence............let it be............ without the hope for sound............just mindful until a sound comes.

When inevitably your mind wanders, notice with curiosity that it has wandered and where it has wandered to. Then, without judgement, bring your attention back to the exercise.

After 10–15 minutes[17] gently bring your awareness back to your surroundings, look around you and maybe stretch. Now it's time for reflection.

Reflection on Exercise 19

It is highly likely that your mind will have wandered from time to time during the exercise above. It may have wandered to things that are going on in your life, things that have happened or things that are likely to happen in the future. Your mind may have wandered to what you heard people saying, questioning whose car door was banging, where a hum was coming from or why your stomach was rumbling. This is of course perfectly normal. The trick isn't to stop your mind wandering, but, when you notice it has, to bring your attention back to the task without judgement.

You may have noticed things slowing down during this exercise and felt more relaxed. Although there is increasing evidence that mindfulness can be helpful to those suffering from sleep problems, the purpose of this particular exercise is not to fall asleep but to create a sense of calm

---

[17]   With any of these exercises, timings are merely guidelines. If you prefer to engage in the exercises for a much longer or shorter time, this is absolutely fine.

awareness in the present moment and provide a space into which we can build self-compassion. This in turn will help build your self-confidence. It is for this reason that I recommend, if possible, that people do the exercise in a sitting position rather than lying down. Of course, if it is helpful to you, you can obviously use this exercise for other purposes also.

After completing each of the mindfulness exercises in this chapter it may be helpful to write down some reflections in your notebook or on your personal practice sheet. In addition, if your mind wandered to particular things during the exercise it may also help to make a note of this. These reflections may provide useful information for future exercises.

Exercise 20: Mindfulness of bodily sensations

Once again, start by finding a location that is, as far as possible, free from major distractions. Somewhere you feel comfortable and can be for 10–15 minutes. If possible sit in an upright posture, with strength in your spine and a sense of openness in your body. It is helpful if you can close your eyes for this exercise, but others may prefer to settle their gaze on a low fixed point.

Notice the sensations in your own body...........notice your breath...........slowly moving in and out...........in and out........... notice the rise and fall of your chest or your belly...........notice the sensations your breath brings with it...........notice your rib-cage expanding then contracting...........notice the temperature of your body...........the warmth in your chest...........notice how your body feels supported...........move your attention round your body, from place to place, and notice how it feels.

When your mind wanders, which it will, gently and curiously notice where it has wandered to and, without judgement, bring your attention back to the exercise.

Sometimes your body will feel tense; you may feel some pain or discomfort. If this is the case just notice the tension, pain or discomfort and then move your attention to another part of your body.

After 10–15 minutes gently bring your awareness back to your surroundings and look around you, maybe having a stretch. Now it's time for reflection.

Reflection on Exercise 20

Because this exercise focuses on the body you may have noticed areas of tension, pain or discomfort. Mindfulness is increasingly found to be a helpful practice for those experiencing pain. If you notice tension, pain or discomfort, be mindful of it, without the need to do anything about it, and then gently and without judgement bring your attention back to the exercise.

For some, concentrating on their breathing or body can be difficult. It may increase anxiety or uncomfortable physical sensations. Although some people find that with practice these sensations decline, if this remains difficult for you, do not spend too long on the exercise. As you can see, there is a wealth of other mindfulness exercises you can try.

Exercise 21: Mindfulness of breathing

In the previous exercise, if you found focusing on your body or the sensation of breathing particularly difficult it is likely that you will find this exercise problematic too. However, many people find focusing on their breathing particularly helpful as a mindfulness practice. This exercise is often associated with a slowing down of your breathing to a comfortable and regular rate. For some it involves noticing how the breath affects one part of the body, such as the belly, the nose or the chest, while for others it involves focusing somewhere else, or on a combination of these.

In later chapters I will discuss how different postures can help you build your self-compassion and self-confidence, but for the purposes of this exercise, if it is possible, I would once again ask you to sit in the way outlined earlier, with a feeling of strength and openness. This is to counteract any tendency you may experience to become so relaxed that you fall asleep.

Start by finding a place that is, as far as possible, free from major distractions. Somewhere you can be for 10–15 minutes. It is helpful if you can close your eyes for this exercise, but some people may prefer to settle their gaze on a low fixed point.

Sit quietly for a moment and bring your attention to your breathing. Be aware of your breath coming into your body............slowly and evenly............maybe you notice the sensation of air coming into and leaving your nose............maybe the rise and fall of your belly............ maybe you are aware of your breath in your chest, rising and falling, or your rib-cage expanding then contracting............move your awareness around your body and, wherever it is most comfortable to notice your breathing, bring your awareness to that area............now just settle and experience your breathing............in and out.

When you are ready, after 10–15 minutes, slowly bring your awareness to your surroundings.

Reflection on Exercise 21

If you find either this or the bodily sensations exercises difficult it may be helpful to engage in one of the anchoring practices (Exercises 22 or 23) alongside it. Alternatively, as such exercises often have a 'slowing down' effect, some people find it helpful to gently repeat in their mind the statement *'slowing down'* as they engage with the exercise, in order to take some of the intensity away. Still others find that they can do the exercise if they pair it with a different activity, such as walking.

Exercise 22: Mindfulness of a visual anchor point

Anchor points can be really helpful for some people in their mindfulness practice. Visual anchor points are something stationary on which you choose to fix your gaze. It usually helps to choose an anchor point approximately 1–2 yards away, and on the floor or low down so that your eyes will be partially closed and less aware of visual distractions.

Your anchor point can be something that you notice in your environment, such as a chair leg, a plant, a piece of kerbstone or a pattern in the flooring. Alternatively it could be something you always use and take with you, such as a ball, a stone, a bag or book.

Once again, start by finding a place that is, as far as possible, free from major distractions. Somewhere you can be for 10–15 minutes. Adjust your posture as you have done previously.

Now identify a fixed anchor point on which you can hold your gaze. It may be something already there or something you place on the ground.

Now observe your anchor point: observe its shape, its edges............ observe its colour and texture............observe how at times it may be in sharp focus, at others it may become fuzzy in places............just observe the object.

When you are ready, gently bring your awareness back to your surroundings and look around you. Now it's time for reflection.

Reflection on Exercise 22

During these exercises your attention might have wandered to any number of things, but while your eyes are open there will be many other sources of distraction. Sometimes these are moving things, such as a leaf fluttering by, a person passing or a bird in flight, but often they are tricks our mind and sight play on us. For example, we may suddenly see a shadow when nothing is moving, may see a 'floater' before our eyes or experience double vision. As with any other occurence that takes our attention away from the exercise, this is perfectly normal. Once again the trick is, when this is noticed, to be mindful that the attention has wandered and bring it back to the practice.

If you are uncomfortable or apprehensive about doing exercises with your eyes closed this is a good exercise to do in preparation for them. Alternatively it can be used as a starting point for future exercises. People often find that they feel more confident about closing their eyes if they know they can open them, at any time, to see a visual anchor point.

Exercise 23: Mindfulness of a tactile anchor point

This exercise is similar to the previous one but instead of using a visual anchor point we are going to use a tactile one. This may be something like a stone, a key ring, a piece of jewellery or a purse or wallet. It is helpful if it is something you can easily hold in one or two hands. It is also important to pick something that isn't associated with difficult emotions that may interfere with the exercise.

Once again start by finding a place that is, as far as possible, free from major distractions. Somewhere you can be for 10–15 minutes.

Now just hold the object in your hand(s) and notice how it feels............ experience its weight............notice the feel of the item............ maybe it's soft, maybe it's hard............maybe it's a combination of the two............notice the temperature of the object and how it feels when you manipulate it in your hands............feel how it is against your skin............continue with the exercise and, when your mind wanders, notice with curiosity where it has wandered to and, without judgement, bring it back to the exercise.

After 10–15 minutes, gently bring your awareness back to your surroundings and look around you. Now it's time for reflection.

Reflection on Exercise 23

Some individuals find that each time they do this exercise they pick a different and novel object. Others find that it is more helpful to do this practice with the same, or similar, object each time. The importance lies not in what you choose to use but whether the object is helpful to you in your practice.

Again this exercise may be used in conjunction with the preceding ones in order to provide the individual with an anchor point, if needed, when the eyes are closed.

The impact our fast-paced lives have on us

It is worth reflecting on the ways that modern life has decreased the opportunities, as well as the motivation, for being 'lost' or absorbed in an activity or moment, without a sense of urgency or need to think about multiple other things. We now live a fast-paced life where many of the activities we used mindfully to engage in are either not valued or not needed.

For example, in days gone by our parents and their parents would absorb themselves in the task of making bread. They would hand-wash clothes, tend the land, darn socks and repair shirts. I am not saying that they never did this with any sense of urgency, worry or upsetting thoughts, but there were simply more opportunities to focus completely on the activity in hand.

Now the pressures of life mean that if I am waiting to see the dentist I am likely to be checking my email; when I peel the vegetables I may also be watching the TV or making a phone call. If I don't practise mindfulness it is easy to let a whole day go by when I have not consciously focused my mind just on the moment.

Whether the object or focus of the mindfulness practice is walking, breathing, washing my hands or drinking coffee, mindfulness allows me and many others to appreciate the moment and s....l....o....w............d....o....w....n.

Exercise 24: Mindful walking

For some individuals, sitting and engaging in these exercises can prove difficult due to pain; others may not be able to find the time to sit still for an exercise or may not see it as a good use of time. Of course, my first comment, if you find yourself in the latter two categories, would be that it is important for you to try and *make* time in order to see for yourself that they are actually extremely helpful in all manner of ways.

If, however, sitting is difficult for you, or you need some persuasion regarding this use of your time or the likely benefits to you of these exercises, I would ask you to engage in the following exercise. Others may simply prefer this form of mindfulness or use it as a helpful addition to their practice.

During the exercise you can either focus on *one* specific element of your experience, such as the sensation of walking or the things you can see, or alternatively you can slowly switch your attention *between* different things, working through the senses: from physical sensations on your skin, to sounds, to things you can see, and maybe to your breathing. Play around with the exercise and find the format that is most helpful to you.

Find somewhere to walk that will be, as far as possible, free from distractions. For example, a busy high street may not be the best place to start. Similarly a local park, at a time when you are likely to see lots of people you know, may prove equally distracting.

Stand for a moment and feel the ground beneath your feet............ feel the strength in your legs supporting you............now as you find yourself walking become aware of what the air feels like on your skin, maybe hot, maybe cold............maybe you can feel the warmth of the sun, droplets of rain or the breeze on your face............notice the sounds as they come and go............let curiosity rather than judgement fill your mind............notice nature around you, the plants, the trees, or look into the sky and see the clouds above, or the pattern of the open sky............ notice smells as they come and go............experience how it feels to walk on the ground.

When you feel ready, gently bring your awareness to the end of the exercise. Now it's time for reflection.

Reflection on Exercise 24

Mindful walking does not mean walking to get somewhere, but walking to be mindful. That said, the exercise can easily be tied into everyday life and for this reason many people find that it becomes a component of their 'self-practice'. You may regularly have to walk a certain route to get somewhere, you may walk your dog or like to engage in physical exercise. If you are tying the exercise into a walk that you *need* to do in any case, make sure you allow yourself extra time so your mind isn't bombarded with associated thoughts.

You may have noted that the other exercises focus on one sense whereas this one focuses on a range of different things e.g. the experience of the ground underfoot, the sensation of the air, the sounds around you. For some the wider focus proves helpful to their practice; for others it is more helpful to attend to one thing at a time. This is a purely personal choice.

Once again, as with all of the exercises, your mind will wander, especially since you have your eyes open and if you are en route to somewhere. But whenever you become mindful that your attention has wandered, notice where it has gone and gently bring it back.

How mindfulness can help with over-striving

In Chapter 3 we looked at the concepts of *value* and *need* achievers plus *growth* seekers and *validation* seekers. Individuals who lack self-confidence can often become so caught up in striving to please others, gain recognition and approval, that they can forget to experience pleasure from an experience in its own right. If you recognize this in yourself, over the next week it may help simply to be mindful of the *process* of working towards a goal or achieving the goal *itself.* Take a breath and bring your complete attention to the moment. If this is helpful it may be incorporated into your daily practice. If you find it difficult it could become the focus of later work. In Chapter 13 we will be looking at the practice of 'savouring', which involves appreciating the moment, and this may help further.

In this exercise there is a greater probability of things being totally disrupted by bumping into someone we know, someone asking us directions or suddenly realizing that the dog has run off (in my case!). However, some people find that being at home is even more distracting than being outside as the doorbell may ring or someone may unexpectedly come into the room. In such instances we can choose to ignore the doorbell, and merely observe it as a sound, but often we cannot ignore interruptions. In such instances it is helpful to acknowledge that we cannot remain undisturbed all the time, respond to the situation and then return to the practice.

Things that may assist you in your practice

During these exercises you are encouraged to close your eyes or lower your gaze. Obviously this makes reading difficult. It may help to make your own recording of the instructions, using a calm, quiet voice. Alternatively, sound files can be found on the Compassionate Mind Foundation website (www.compassionatemind.co.uk). As you become more familiar with the exercises it is likely that you will be able to practise them from memory.

Problem-solving Around Common Difficulties With These Exercises

- What to do about recurring thoughts and images

As I have mentioned previously, during any exercise or practice our attention will be drawn towards any number of things. Sometimes it will be a sound and we may start to wonder where it came from, or we may start to think about what we are going to have for dinner, or reflect on what a nice day it was yesterday. However, sometimes we may notice that our minds repeatedly go to a specific situation, past, present or future, a particular worry or rumination.

If you have this experience it may be helpful to make this the focus of some of the later exercises covered in this book. But for the time being maybe just jot down the difficulties you are having. You can then refer back to them later on.

• What to do if you feel intense emotions

People sometimes experience intense emotions when they practise mindfulness – it is as though the process clears a space into which emotions that have been hidden, bottled up or suppressed, move. This makes sense because most people will be used to keeping themselves or their minds busy in order not to have to deal with more difficult things. If your emotions are manageable then just view them with curiosity and non-judgement and return to the exercise. Other people find that any of the anchoring practices may help here. If, however, the emotions feel more intense, making your practice difficult to return to, maybe just allow yourself to sit with the emotion for a while and experience it. Strong emotions can feel frightening and uncomfortable, but they do subside. Often, allowing ourselves to experience intense emotions, such as sadness and anger, and then feeling them fade away, can actually be a healing process.

Again, you may find some of the later exercises helpful in this respect so it may be your choice to move on to these now instead of working straight through the book, though it would be a good idea to return to this section at a later date.

• What if you really can't settle to do the exercise because your mind is racing?

I hope that during these exercises, when you become aware of intrusive thoughts, images or bodily sensations, you will simply reflect that your mind has switched focus and then bring it back to the exercise. However, we all have times when mindfulness and similar practices become more difficult. Usually these experiences are associated with strong emotions which seem to get in the way. Funnily enough, these are often the times we most need to practise.

At the start of the book I mentioned that it is best to start this work when things are relatively 'easy' for you. However, if you find that you are some way into your practice and this happens, or alternatively there never *is* an easy time, the following suggestions may be helpful.

1. Engage in the exercise, accepting without criticism that our brains have a 'mind of their own' that we simply cannot control absolutely.

2. If you are criticizing yourself or becoming frustrated, treat this in the same way, observing it and then returning to the exercise.

3. Engage with the exercise fleetingly, despite the distractions. You may be surprised to find just how helpful even snatched moments can be.

4. Write down the things that are on your mind before you begin, and then attempt to leave those things behind on the paper while you do the exercise. It is often interesting how much easier it is to think things through after a mindfulness practice.

5. It may be that some of the later exercises will be of greater benefit to you, so move on to those.

How to Develop Your Own Mindfulness 'Self-practice'

As you try out the above exercises it is likely that you will find ones that are good for you and others that are less so. I would encourage you to practise regularly those exercises that you find most helpful, trying them on for size, with your future 'self-practice' in mind. Practising them for a week or so before continuing with the rest of this book may be helpful. If, however, you are keen not to have a break, you can continue to practise them alongside your further reading.

Once you have a *feel* for what mindfulness is, you can begin to play around with how you introduce it to other areas of your life as well. Here are some examples:

- Michelle Cree, who is a clinical psychologist working with pregnant women and new mothers , suggests *mindful hand washing* as a way of regularly building mindfulness into a busy day. The exercise involves being mindful of the feel of water on the skin, the sound of running water and the smell of soap.

- Susan Albers, in her 2006 book *Mindful Eating*, advocates using mindfulness in a number of ways in relation to food. Modern life means that we often eat whilst sitting in front of the TV or 'on the go', all of which can prevent us really experiencing the texture, taste and smell of our food. Mindful attention to the food we eat can help us appreciate it more and lead to a better relationship with it, and with ourselves.

- In the CFT groups I run I encourage people to practise mindfulness whenever they drink a cup of tea or coffee. Drinking mindfully is a very different experience from drinking while sitting in front of a computer screen or watching TV. People most commonly report that in practising mindful drinking their brain gets a break from the worries and ruminations that occupy their minds. It is also a good reminder to integrate other aspects of the therapy into their everyday lives.

In short, mindfulness practice can be done for long or short intervals, inside or outside, as part of another activity or as an activity in its own right, in a busy or peaceful place, day or night.

Finally, while some may find that it is easy to motivate themselves to do 10–15 minutes of mindfulness practice per day, others find Post-it notes on the fridge or something like a pebble in their pocket remind them to engage in self-practice. In the mindfulness in schools initiative (see www.mindfulnessinschools.org for further information) high-school children 'buddy up' and randomly text each other once a day the message '.b'. This stands for 'Stop ... breathe'. Participants report this to be a really effective way of bringing mindfulness into their everyday lives. Maybe you can ask a friend or relative to practise mindfulness also, and then you can experiment with supporting each other through text messages.

As with any of these exercises, what is important is finding something that works for you.

Conclusions

Mindfulness practices have been found by many to be hugely beneficial in their own right, and hopefully this will be the case for you. If you wish to pursue mindfulness practice further there are many excellent books you may wish to read, a number of which are listed in the Further Reading section on page 265.

In the compassionate mind approach, we encourage you to engage in some form of mindfulness, to provide you with a space or foundation on which you can build self-compassion and through this develop your self-confidence.

8 Further Preparation for Compassion

The practice of mindfulness outlined in the previous chapter aims to bring you to a state of *calm awareness*, which has curiosity and non-judgement. Mindfulness practice brings awareness to the present moment and, when we notice that our attention has been drawn to something else, observes where it has gone and gently returns it to the practice.

Although not a direct aim of mindfulness, individuals often report feeling a sense of *warmth, contentment* or *soothing* during their mindfulness practice. It is this feeling that we will now attempt to nurture directly.

Developing Your Soothing System

We will now concentrate on two exercises. The first is a soothing rhythm breathing exercise which aims to evoke and develop your own natural capacity for self-soothing. As with any of the exercises, if you find it difficult, try for a little while but, ultimately, do not continue with anything that seems to have an adverse effect on you, i.e. resulting in difficult emotions rather than a soothing and calming experience. There are a large number of exercises in this book that you can try instead. Remember, in the compassionate mind approach, you need not 'succeed' in one exercise before you move on to the next.

The second exercise uses imagery as a means of creating a sensory experience, and the aim is to develop a personal *place of contentment* created in your own mind. Again, if this is difficult for you there are some further ideas that may help you later in the chapter.

Both exercises are listed on the personal practice summary sheet on page xxviii of the Preface. It may be helpful to use this, as well as your notebook, to record your reflections.

Exercise 25: Soothing rhythm breathing

Soothing rhythm breathing is a specific breathing practice that aims to switch on and develop your soothing system. The exercise is designed to help you find *your own* soothing rhythm. For many this often involves slowing your breathing to a comfortable, deep and regular rate. Unlike some forms of relaxation training, it does not require you to adopt a specific pace – rather it is about finding a pace that is right for you. It also includes an element of mindfulness. As such, during this exercise, when you notice your awareness has moved to something else, be mindful of where it has gone and gently bring it back to your breathing.

People focus on different things to help them concentrate during this exercise. Some concentrate on the nostrils, others on the chest or rib-cage, or on counting breaths in, pausing and then counting them out, or on a combination of these things. You may already have an idea of what is helpful for you based on the mindfulness of breathing exercise in the previous chapter, but this exercise will help you explore this further.

Once again, start by finding a place that is, as far as possible, free from major distractions. Somewhere you can be for 10–15 minutes. If you can, sit with an upright posture, feet on the floor approximately hip-distance apart, hands gently resting on your lap. Feel a strength in your spine, yet a relaxation in your body and a sense of openness. It is helpful if you can close your eyes for this exercise, but some people may prefer to settle their gaze on a low fixed point.

Sit quietly for a moment and bring your attention to your breathing............noticing the air going in and out through your nose............ maybe being aware of the rise and fall of your belly............gradually rising and slowly falling............maybe being aware of your chest rising and falling............aware of your rib-cage expanding then contracting............It may help to breathe in to your own count of three............pausing and then exhaling, again to a count of three............finding a breathing pattern that, for you, seems to be your own soothing, comforting rhythm.

Maybe experimenting a little with your breathing............breathing a little faster and then a little slower, and noticing the difference in how your body feels............Once you have found a soothing rhythm, experience it for a few minutes............allowing the air to come into your body slowly and evenly, then leave it............slowly and evenly, in a breathing rhythm that is soothing for you.

When you are ready, gently bring your awareness to the end of the exercise, becoming more aware of your physical environment. Now it is time for reflection.

Using your sense of smell to assist you

Some people find the soothing breathing rhythm exercise difficult, if not virtually impossible. However, if the exercise is paired with a smell they find soothing, this can sometimes be extremely helpful. The smell could be that of a perfume or aftershave, a soap, moisturizer, essential oil or anything that you find *soothing*. Sometimes it can be a scent with no associations for you, other times it is something that has positive memories attached to it. There is good reason why people find this helpful. Our olfactory (smell) receptors 'fast track' to the limbic system, thought to be the home of emotion. Unpleasant smells can therefore very quickly trigger our threat system and a fast-acting emotional experience of anxiety, anger or repulsion. In contrast, pleasant smells can have a very fast-acting *positive* emotional response, bringing 'on-line' our contentment and soothing system, thereby creating a sense of soothing.

Reflection on Exercise 25

For many, the soothing rhythm breathing exercise feels quite different to the mindfulness of breathing exercise in the last chapter. This is because in the soothing rhythm exercise you are focusing on bring-ing your soothing system 'on-line' – in contrast to previous exercises where the primary aim is to bring calm awareness of the moment as it occurs.

If you were able to find your own soothing breathing rhythm you may have noticed that this affects the way you experience thoughts and images that pop into your mind.

It is important to point out here that we are not aiming to *achieve* any specific emotional or physical state in this exercise. Instead it is designed to help you switch on your soothing system. Once this is brought *on-line* it is likely that your emotional or physical state will alter *as a consequence*, but this is not the primary aim. Remember, it's not the destination but the journey that counts. Spend too long thinking about a desired outcome and you will disrupt the practice.

As with the mindfulness exercises, once you have experienced and prac-tised using your soothing breathing rhythm you can then develop your own self-practice. You may, for example, choose to engage with your soothing rhythm breathing at certain set times in the week. You may decide to practise it while walking, during a coffee break or in the shower or bath.

Exercise 26: Finding your place of contentment

The purpose of this exercise is to evoke a sense of contentment. As with the soothing rhythm breathing exercise this will then be used as a further platform on which to build your self-compassion and self-confidence. Here imagery is used to create a broader sensory experience. Your own place of contentment may be an idealized version of somewhere that is real, or somewhere that is purely imaginary. Alternatively it may be a combination of different places. It is not accessible to the things that threaten us, but is devoid of such things. It is a place that always welcomes you.

A note about your place of contentment

For some, a place of contentment is different from a 'safe place', although both can evoke very similar sensory experiences. Within this book I intentionally do not use classic 'safe-place' imagery, preferring instead to use the term 'place of contentment', as the latter option seems less fraught with opportunity for the threat system to muscle in on the experience. More specifically, some people report that use of the term 'safe' conjures up contradictory elements of threat in their image. Others report that they can only experience a feeling of being 'safe' in the context of threat – that which they are safe from – therefore inadvertently evoking the threat system. As such, people sometimes report a menacing element to a 'safe place', maybe on the fringes, seeing or sensing another person or the critical part of themselves.

I do, however, use the term, and the practice, 'safe place' at times. For some, creating a 'safe place', that has defences against threat, may be a necessary stepping stone to evoking our sense of contentment. For example, someone may initially imagine themselves in a 'safe place' cocooned from threat by a magical blanket or a force field. Others imagine that they are in a bunker thirty feet underground. It is hoped that with time and practice the experience will evolve to one where there is no need for such precautions, just a place that is welcoming and devoid of all threats. As with any of these exercises, there is no right and wrong way of doing things. What is important is finding something that works for you and brings your own soothing system 'on-line'.

Once again, this exercise includes an element of mindfulness. Remember, when you become mindful that your awareness has moved to something else, notice where it has gone and gently bring it back to the exercise.

While some people find it helpful to embark on this exercise in a spirit of curiosity as to where they will end up, others find it helpful to do some preparation around an initial image they will begin to explore *from*. Still others find that it is helpful for them to think about what kind of place they are going to steer their mind towards. If you think it may be beneficial for you, take some time to think about the types of place in which you feel, or have felt, a sense of contentment. Maybe there was a particular picture you felt was warm and inviting. Places often generated by people are images of a beach, a wood or of being in a warm house in front of an open fire. Preparatory questions you may ask yourself are whether you are outside or inside? What smells and sounds are there around you? Can you hear the birds, the wind in the trees or a crackling fire? Can you smell burning wood, freshly cut grass, or water gently lapping against the sides of a boat or on the shore? Would you be looking out from a beach hut or cabin on to an expanse of ocean or woodland? What would the weather be like? What colours would there be around you?

If your mind goes to a real place, it may be helpful to ask yourself whether that place has any negative connotations attached to it. For example, a childhood bedroom may seem, for some, to be an ideal spot to think about as a place of contentment – but if it was somewhere where you felt uncomfortable at times it may also conjure up difficult memories and emotions that would distract you from the purpose of this exercise. You could, however, pick aspects of the room, things that made you feel secure and content, but blend them with other things. Like a designer, you can pick and choose how you want the place to look. Remember, this is your idealized place.

It is important to find something that works for you personally. It is also true that what works for you in one situation may not in another, so play around with it, finding something that is right for you at that moment in time.

Once again, start by finding a place that is, as far as possible, free from distractions. Somewhere you can be peacefully for 10–15 minutes. Seat yourself comfortably, feeling strength in your spine yet relaxation in your body and a sense of openness. It is helpful if you can close your eyes for this exercise, but some may prefer to settle their gaze on a low fixed point.

Before this exercise, if you find it helpful, start by using your soothing rhythm breathing. Alternatively use one of the other mindfulness practices from Chapter 7 to create a sense of calm awareness. Or you may prefer to go straight into the exercise.

Ideas to help with imagery

While some people find it very easy to conjure up images, it is quite normal for others to find this difficult. If this is the case for you, here are a few things that other people have used to help them:

- Imagine a colour around you, maybe in the form of a mist, maybe a blanket

- Find a picture, either a photo or a drawing or painting, that you can focus on and feel yourself into

- Imagine a channel of warm light flowing into and out of your body, from the crown of your head to the tips of your toes

- Find a piece of soothing music that gives you a sense of contentment

- Experiment with different smells and see if any of them can evoke a sense of contentment

There are no rights and wrongs in the compassionate mind approach. What is important is gaining a sense of experience and then developing it further.

When you feel ready, begin to create a place in your mind............a place in which you can experience a sense of contentment and calmness............you may be focusing on a picture or an image you have thought about previously........you could simply be waiting to see where your mind takes you.

As you begin to develop a fleeting impression of what the place will be like, you will now explore what your senses experience in this place............What can you see?............Maybe objects, maybe vegetation or animals, maybe an expanse of water or a beach............ What sorts of colours can you see?............Now, what sounds can you hear?............Maybe the rustling of leaves, a breeze, water............ maybe the faint sound of music, muffled noises, the distant sound of children laughing, birds singing............How does the air feel?............ Is it warm or cold?............Do you feel the sun on your skin?............

Are there any smells that you notice?............Maybe the scent of grass or the saltiness of the ocean............maybe a waft of scent or the smell of bread............Think about your place of contentment and explore it with all your senses............maybe staying with one in particular for a while if you find it soothing.

Your wandering mind will take your attention away from this place............When you become mindful that it has wandered, notice where it has moved to and gently return your attention to that part of the experience you find most associated with a sense of contentment, then continue.

Imagine yourself in the image............what is supporting your body?............Maybe the ground is contoured perfectly against it............maybe you are sitting on a cool rock, a cosy bed or warm sand ....Become aware of your own warm facial expression, maybe a half-smile…a content gaze.

Now, experience the knowledge that this place welcomes you............ Its sole purpose is to help *you* experience a sense of contentment and warmth............It is in harmony with you.

After engaging in this exercise and experiencing it for 10–15 minutes, gently bring it to an end and focus your awareness back on your physical environment.

Reflection on Exercise 26

It may be that you will need to do this exercise a number of times before a helpful image comes to mind. Alternatively you may try using some of the aids other people have found helpful when developing their own places, which are listed in the Imagery text box on page 124.

Your 'place of contentment' is personal to you and therefore you can adapt it as your needs change – it is not fixed.

Even when people settle on a particular image or experience, many of them report that they appreciate a *fluidity* to it, in contrast to its remaining static, like a photo. It would seem that this prevents them from growing over-familiar with their place of contentment and losing the richness of the experience over time.

Whereas some people do not object to hearing background sounds during these exercises, others find this more difficult. What is important is what evokes a sense of contentment in you. A further thing that people sometimes find difficult is the idea that the place 'welcomes' you. In Compassion Focused Therapy we think that this is an important component of the practice (but not essential) as, for many, it enhances the stimulation of your soothing system. Remember, we can soothe ourselves but we can also be soothed by others. As your place welcomes you it becomes a soothing agent.

As noted at the start of this exercise you are being encouraged, wherever possible, to adopt a posture that has strength and openness in it. This is especially important as many people find that they can become extremely relaxed, to the point of falling asleep, during this exercise. Later, it may be of benefit to use this exercise as a method to help you sleep. However, here we will be using it as a foundation for other things that will empower you and build your self-confidence – and if you are going to do this, it helps to remain alert and strong rather than sleepy!

Conclusions

This chapter has introduced to your mindfulness practice two further exercises that are designed specifically to help you access your soothing system. Mindfulness in this instance is the means by which we refocus on the practice, rather than the practice itself. (But of course you may also wish to explore other aspects of mindfulness.)

Although these exercises involve quite a lot of 'doing', you may be itching or agitating to 'do more' specifically to build your self-confidence. This may be your drive system at play. It is important to emphasize, however, that this work is likely to impact on your self-confidence. Mindfulness can help you *disengage* from your threat system and difficult thoughts, images and emotions, while your *soothing rhythm breathing* and the *place of contentment* practice bring your soothing system *on-line* to help you regulate or *tone down* your threat system.

9 Developing Your Compassionate Mind

Having looked at self-confidence in some detail, and made a case for building it, the evolutionary origins of our emotional states, and how these relate to self-confidence, were explained. After examining the effects of self-undermining and how self-compassion may help with this, you were then encouraged to think about your own situation – both the events that led you to the point where you are now, and the things that maintain your situation – by means of a *formulation* or diagrammatic representation. This hopefully helped address any self-criticism you may experience. It should also have given you an indication of the areas of your life that it may be beneficial for you to address.

The focus of this chapter is on developing your compassionate mind or mindset and, more specifically, the key dimension of *self*-compassion. We will do this through a number of different imagery exercises (though it is worth noting that for some the experience will be more sensory than visual). While some exercises offer different approaches to achieving the same thing, others are distinct. It is hoped that practising a combination of these will enable you to build up the different aspects of your compassionate mind, and in particular self-compassion.

Through the compassionate mindset we can discover new ways of thinking about things, new motivations, new behaviours and more pleasurable emotions. This mindset will also help us *tone down* the threat system that is associated with experiences such as anxiety, anger and habitual undermining of ourselves.

The importance of facial expressions and posture

Our facial expressions and posture can have a profound effect on the way we feel and how others perceive us. A number of studies have demonstrated that we can consciously manipulate such things to good effect. For example, one study demonstrated that it was possible to manipulate how funny participants found cartoons by instructing them to do one of two things. While looking at the images, the first group was told to hold a pencil between their teeth, ensuring that it did not touch their lips. The second group were told to hold the pencil in their mouth, without it touching their teeth. The former group 'enjoyed' or found the cartoons funnier than the second group. This was attributed to the smile that was elicited by the first facial position (using teeth only). We also know that people who have a smile on their face are considered, by others, to be warmer and more approachable. Therefore smiling can make us enjoy things more *and* make us more likely to have positive interactions with others.

Similarly, and something that has been practised by 'method actors' for decades, we can manipulate our posture as a way of evoking particular emotions. Posture can also influence the way we think, what we pay attention to and how our body feels. For example, if you were to walk down the street with your head held low, your spine curved, dragging your feet and lowering your gaze, it is likely to have an impact on your mood, your thoughts and how you feel physically. However, if you were to walk with strength in your spine, lowering your shoulders, with an inquisitive gaze and a bounce in your step, it is likely that your mood will reflect this, and your thoughts are likely to be more positive. You are also likely to feel better physically. If this posture were combined with an open and warm facial expression, it is likely that you would be seen by others as more approachable.

All of this is so important because sometimes if we wait to do something until we *feel* like it, we can be waiting a long time. Sometimes it is about doing something despite not *feeling like it* and using the manipulation of our posture and facial expression to help us do it – it's not about kidding yourself but about giving yourself a helping hand.

Developing Different Aspects of Your Compassionate Mind or Mindset

It is intended that the following exercises will form the basis of your future self-practice, and that you will use them throughout the rest of your life to enhance your own well-being. Since you will be returning to them frequently, it may be worthwhile spending some time recording yourself reading them aloud, so that you can follow them with minimal disturbance. Alternatively sound files of each of these exercises can be found on the compassionate mind website (www.compassionatemind. co.uk).

What is self-compassion?

In Chapter 5 we discovered that compassion is a mentality or a mindset that has certain attributes, such as empathy, non-judgement and distress tolerance, all practised in the context of *warmth*. Self-compassion involves experiencing these things in relation to yourself and your experiences. In addition, in some of the exercises in this chapter you will be encouraged to employ the following qualities:

Wisdom: The wisdom of self-compassion tells us that where we find ourselves today is *not our fault*. Our complicated brains are the product of evolution and are equipped with a need for nurturing, have a 'better safe than sorry' default setting, and are home to all manner of conflicting emotions and drives. Our brains are further shaped by experiences throughout our lives, and all of this leads us to behave, think and feel in certain ways.

Strength, fortitude and courage: These qualities give us an inner strength and confidence to face the things we need to face, often despite our threat system urging us to avoid or ignore a perceived danger. If we are self-compassionate, we can place ourselves in situations knowing that, no matter what, we will be OK.

Responsibility: This involves recognizing that, although something is 'not our fault', we need to make a commitment to ourselves, and sometimes others, to do our best to resolve the issue. Together with wisdom, strength and warmth, responsibility helps us face the things we need to address, rather than turn away.

Many people initially report that they find it much easier to work on these qualities of self-compassion when they are finding other attributes, such as sympathy and empathy, difficult to practise. So, if certain components of compassion are hard for you at first, start with what is easy and develop things from there.

Exercise 27: Being deeply compassionate

This exercise will help you explore and develop an idea of what compassion *feels* like within your *mind and body*. You will be encouraged to explore a range of different qualities in turn, paying attention to how these feel in your mind and then how they feel in your body. Some people may find this easy while others may struggle and require additional practice. For the purposes of this exercise it doesn't matter if you feel you *actually* possess these qualities or not.

During this exercise it may be helpful for you to think of yourself as an actor. Actors aren't required to have personal experience of everything they represent, but instead to 'try on' the experience and embody it. While 'getting into character' they stimulate certain qualities in their mind and body. They are then able to 'inhabit' the character and 'become' the person they are attempting to portray. Try and approach this exercise in the same way.

Before you begin, start by finding a place that is, as far as possible, free from distractions. Somewhere you can be for 10–15 minutes. Sit in a relaxed, open posture with *strength* or *alertness* to it. It is helpful if you can close your eyes for this exercise, but others may prefer to settle their gaze on a low fixed point.

If the practices were helpful to you previously, embark upon all or any of the exercises in this chapter by first using your soothing rhythm breathing or 'place of contentment' exercise. Alternatively, use one of the mindfulness practices to create a sense of calm awareness, or else simply go straight into the exercise once your mind and body are settled. Remember, there are no rights and wrongs in the compassionate mind approach.

Now imagine you are a deeply compassionate person............experience what it feels like............How does it feel in your mind and in your body?..........Maybe you find that you sit differently or experience your body differently............maybe your facial expression changes when you step into the role of a deeply compassionate person?..........It may be that this does not come automatically and you need to change your posture or your expression intentionally............This is OK............What is important is that you get a sense of what it feels like to be a deeply compassionate person.

Wisdom tells us that we all just find ourselves here..........we are the product of our genes and our nurture............this is not our fault............it is something we have no control over............for a moment, experience how it feels, in your mind and in your body, to know this.

Now, feeling strength............fortitude............courage in your mind ....how does that feel now in your body?............Maybe you find that you sit differently or experience your body differently............ maybe it helps to adjust your posture in order to help yourself feel these things.

Now, with the experience of wisdom, strength, fortitude and courage, experience the quality of warmth............how does that feel in your mind?............How does it feel in your body?............Imagine yourself speaking to someone and hearing the warm tone of your voice.

Experience within your mind how it feels to hold a commitment to address things in a compassionate way............now feel it within your body............a motivation to face difficulties and increase well-being through compassion.

After about 10–15 minutes gently bring your awareness to the end of the exercise, becoming more aware of your physical environment. Now it's time for reflection.

Settling your mind and body

In the previous chapters you were encouraged to explore mindfulness, soothing rhythm breathing and a place of contentment. Through the process of engaging with such exercises it is likely that you developed your own way of settling your mind and body before you began. As such, when prompted, engage in those things that you find to be helpful.

Reflection on Exercise 27

As this is the first exercise that looks specifically at the experience of compassion, you may find it challenging and require further practice before you feel you can recognize the feeling within your mind and body.

Although the compassionate mind approach aims to create a compassionate mindset, it also pays particular attention to the associated physical sensations because mind and body are closely connected. Our mindset affects the way we feel physically. For example, if we are in a threat mindset our stomachs may churn, we may feel sick, tense, experience a sensation of pins and needles or chest pain. The focus of our attention may turn to the way our body is feeling, and this may further increase the sense of threat. By contrast, in a compassionate mindset we are likely to feel a sense of relaxed alertness, warmth and strength, in both mind and body. It is hoped that paying equal attention to both will create an enhanced sense of compassion.

You may have found that your posture and expression changed slightly during the exercise – or you may consciously have tried to change them. Some people report that with a change of posture they gain an increased sense of relaxation and warmth, together with more strength and alertness. Others state that they find they sit up straighter and develop a more relaxed facial expression, maybe with a half-smile or a sense of warmth in their eyes (even if they are closed).

Exercise 28: Re-experiencing your own compassion

Before doing this exercise it may be helpful to spend a little time bringing to mind an occasion when you felt a sense of compassion and/or acted in a compassionate way. Try not to concentrate on a situation that could be charged with very strong emotions as this may raise all sorts of confusing feelings within you. Instead start with something that is neither charged with strong emotions nor devoid of them. Usually people find that it is easiest to think about a situation where they experienced compassion being directed towards someone else than it is to recall it being directed towards themselves. Maybe you can remember a time when you helped someone in need: a child that had hurt itself, or someone who was going through a difficult time.

Find a place where you can be for 10–15 minutes that is, as far as possible, free from distractions. Sit in a relaxed, open posture that has *strength* or *alertness* in it. Close your eyes or settle your gaze on a low fixed point.

Now bring to mind a time when you felt compassion towards someone or acted in a compassionate way............recalling the event and thinking yourself into the situation............how do you experience compassion in your mind?............How does it feel in your body?............Maybe you feel a sense of warmth, of strength, or an urge to move towards the individual............What facial expression does it evoke?............What posture does it move you into?............If you spoke, what would your tone of voice be like?

Experiencing the sense of caring for the other person's well-being............ being moved by that person's experience............being motivated to do what you believe will help them............being able to witness and toler-ate their distress, not turn away............being sensitive to that person without judging them............feeling a strong motivation to alleviate their distress.

After about 10–15 minutes, gently bring an end to the exercise and become more aware of your physical environment.

Reflection on Exercise 28

For some, this exercise can be an extremely powerful way of highlighting their own natural compassion. It can also help them to analyse the experience of compassion. We often view the outcome of a situation as the only part of it worth noting. By recalling all the different elements of this exercise, you can give yourself a better and more in-depth understanding of how the process of compassion *feels*.

If you were recalling an emotionally charged situation, it may stimulate thoughts in you of what happened previously or subsequently. If this is the case, either attempt to focus on the compassionate component and be mindful of when your mind wanders to other things, or else try the exercise again while recalling a different experience, one that is less clouded by other associations.

You may wonder why we are doing this exercise as you yourself have no problem feeling compassionate towards others. Indeed many people find that they fall into the trap of being so compassionate to others that it is to their own detriment. However, the purpose of this exercise is not to develop in you compassion for others, but to let you explore how compassion *feels* through reflecting on the experience of compassion for others. This will help later when you start to develop self-compassion.

Exercise 29: The ideal compassionate self

Find a place where you can be for 10–15 minutes that is, as far as possible, free from distractions. Sit in a relaxed, open posture that has *strength* or *alertness* in it. Close your eyes or settle your gaze on a low fixed point.

Now for a moment imagine that a self-supporting or compassionate part of you could be thought of as a person............spend a few moments imagining and experiencing this............Now imagine becoming that person............move into and assume the role just as an actor may step into a part...............a compassionate ideal............devoid of human preoccupations and conflicts.

How does this feel in the body?............How do you experience it in your mind?............What is the posture of the ideal compassionate self? ....What is the facial expression?............If you were able to look at your ideal compassionate self, what would it look like? ....Old or young?............Large or small?............Are there colours or particular smells that come to mind associated with this image?............Do you feel a sense of warmth?

In the role of the ideal compassionate self, experience a pure sensation of caring for well-being............experiencing sympathy............ empathy............tolerance of distress............being sensitive and non-judgemental............Feel the wisdom of the ideal compassionate self............the warmth............the strength and courage............feel the commitment to resolving difficulties and moving towards well-being.

After 10–15 minutes gently bring an end to the exercise and become more aware of your physical environment.

Reflection on Exercise 29

It is important to remember that the purpose of this exercise is to assume the role of an 'ideal' compassionate self. No human individual can be free from feelings of conflict, struggling and 'failing', because these are what *make* us human. Drives and desires, 'better safe than sorry' thinking, our physical needs, and all manner of other things constantly compete for attention within our minds and bodies. We may wish to maintain the qualities of compassion but find it impossible. However, we can develop and enhance the capacity to be compassionate towards ourselves, and all of the things that make us human, with practice.

You may have noticed the ideal compassionate self as being older than you, in some way softer, you may have felt a sense of warmth and ease in their presence.

As with any of these exercises, when you notice your mind has wandered, note where it has been drawn to and then gently and warmly bring it back to the exercise.

Exercise 30: Evoking a memory of compassion from others

In Chapter 2 I outlined how, in an ideal world, we learn to be soothing to ourselves through initially receiving soothing from others. In other words, a child who has been regularly soothed by a parent, over time learns to internalize this and eventually is able to do it for itself. This does not mean that they no longer experience strong reactions to difficult events, but it does mean that they can eventually calm themselves down, accept help from others, and ultimately feel better about a situation over time.

But in some people this ability to soothe themselves is underdeveloped. Whether this is true for you, or if you simply need to maintain or enhance your ability to self-soothe, the following exercise may be of benefit to you.

In preparation for the exercise, bring to mind the memory of an occasion when someone was there for you. They knew exactly what you needed at the time, be it a hug, a sympathetic ear when you wanted to talk or rant, or maybe they simply supported you by being present. A time when someone was sensitive to your distress, strong, non-judgemental, and had your well-being at heart. A time when you felt a deep sense of connection with someone.

As with the other exercises in this chapter, try not to pick a memory that is closely linked to a very strong or difficult emotion. This can happen if we think about, for example, someone who has since died or whom we no longer see, or about a really distressing time in our lives – something that is always likely to arouse strong emotion in us. This is not to say that it may not be helpful, at some future time, to reflect on such events, but for the purposes of this exercise it is better to start with something easier.

Find a place where you can be for 10–15 minutes that is, as far as possible, free from distractions. Sit in a relaxed, open posture that has *strength* or *alertness* in it. Close your eyes or settle your gaze on a low fixed point.

Now bring to mind an experience when you felt a deep sense of connection with someone............A time when you were struggling and they were compassionate towards you............they knew exactly what you needed and did it.................maybe they were sympathetic and non-judgemental...........wise and strong...........sensitive to your situation and tolerant of your distress.

Bring to mind their facial expression and maybe their posture........... bring to mind the environment you were in and what it looked like...........what it smelt like............bring to mind the sounds around you, maybe the tone of their voice............If they hugged you, what did it feel like?............If they touched your arm or gave you a reassuring nod, how did that feel?............Recall how somebody's compassion for you felt............in both your mind and your body.

Spend time evoking the memory and experiencing it. After a while gently bring an end to the exercise and become more aware of your physical environment.

Reflection on Exercise 30

There is no universal pattern of compassionate behaviour. For some, in the moment, it's a hug and/or a compassionate gaze in which you know that the individual is there for you; for others it's having their mind taken away from a difficult time, but once again with the knowledge that the person is motivated by your best interests. For most people it is a mixture of these things at different times. What is common, however, is the sensation of the other person doing for you exactly what you need at that time.

Memories of real events can be extremely powerful in evoking a sense of connectedness to others, a sense of not being on your own. Unfortunately, depression and anxiety can sometimes make it difficult for us to bring to mind such positive memories; instead we recall anxiety-provoking or depressing events. For others there may simply be a lack of positive memories to call upon. If either of these cases applies to you it may help to think back to whether there was once a friend at school, a kindly teacher or a supportive colleague. It need not be someone you knew for a long time.

If you can find one positive memory, and use this exercise in conjunction with it, you may find that it helps you recall others. Such memories may pop into your mind during or after you have finished the exercise or in the days afterwards. If this is the case for you, jot down any new memories so you can use them later.

Whether such a memory was easily recalled or proved to be more difficult, if you found this exercise helpful it may be useful to repeat it using additional memories as well.

In the next two exercises we will first turn compassion outwards, towards others, and then towards someone who struggles with self-confidence. This will be a further stepping stone to learning to be compassionate towards yourself and your own situation.

Exercise 31: Turning compassion outwards

Ultimately you are hoping to develop self-compassion for your own struggles with self-confidence, as an antidote to self-criticism and a source of future strength and resilience. From this mindset you can then coach yourself in the building of your self-confidence like an encouraging, supportive teacher.

In preparation for this exercise, bring to mind someone you care about who is going through some form of difficulty at the moment. It could be a friend, relative or partner. Use this person as the focus of your compassion. Once again, be careful not to think about someone who is likely to bring up other difficult emotions, such as someone you can no longer be with or someone who is experiencing acute difficulties at the moment.

Find a place where you can be for 10–15 minutes that is, as far as possible, free from distractions. Sit in a relaxed, open posture that has *strength* or *alertness* in it. Close your eyes or settle your gaze on a low fixed point.

Reminding yourself of the compassionate mind's attributes and qualities............experience a pure sense of care for well-being............ sympathy............empathy............tolerance of distress............ sensitivity and non-judgement............Feel the wisdom of your compassionate mind............the warmth............the strength and courage............Feel the commitment to resolve difficulties and move towards well-being............feel these qualities in both your mind and your body.

Now bringing to mind the person you wish to direct compassion towards............experience your own compassion towards them............experience a pure sense of care for their well-being............ sympathy and empathy............tolerance of distress............sensitivity and non-judgement............Feel the wisdom of your compassionate mind............the warmth............the strength and courage............feel the commitment to help to resolve their difficulties and let them move towards well-being............Feel these qualities in both your mind and your body.

When you are ready, gently bring an end to the exercise and become more aware of your physical environment.

Reflection on Exercise 31

People often find during this exercise that their minds will wander with thoughts of, for example, when they are going to see this particular person next, what they did last time they saw them, or what they are doing now. This is perfectly normal. What is important is noticing when your mind has wandered from the exercise, being mindful of where it has gone to and gently bringing it back.

People performing this exercise often experience a heightened sense of emotion. This is because cells in our brain named 'mirror neurons' are firing, and giving us a strong sense of how the other person must be feeling as well as a sense of connectedness to them. This is why you are encouraged, at least initially, to engage in this exercise by focusing on someone who is not in acute distress.

Once you have practised compassion for someone you care about in this more general way, you can then attempt to develop compassion specifically towards those who struggle in a similar way to you. This is the focus of the next exercise.

Exercise 32: Compassion for those who lack self-confidence

This exercise will involve directing your compassionate mind or mindset towards people who may be similar to you in that they lack self-confidence.

In preparation for this exercise think about someone whom you think lacks self-confidence. It may be a person you know well, someone you know merely by sight or someone in the public eye. You may choose someone who lacks self-confidence in every area of their life or in just one area, and to a greater or a lesser extent.

Find a place where you can be for 10–15 minutes that is, as far as possible, free from distractions. Sit in a relaxed, open posture that has *strength* or *alertness* in it. Close your eyes or settle your gaze on a low fixed point.

Reminding yourself of the compassionate mind's qualities............experience a pure sense of care for well-being............sympathy............ empathy............tolerance of distress............sensitivity and non-judgement............Feel the wisdom of your compassionate mind............the warmth............the strength and courage............Feel the commitment to resolve difficulties and move towards well-being............Feel these qualities in both your mind and your body.

Now bring to mind a person who is lacking in self-confidence and direct those compassionate qualities towards them ....consider the things that may have contributed towards their difficulties............consider the effort they need to put into getting through situations others seem to find easy............Consider the impact their lack of self-confidence has on them............The things they have and haven't done............the traps they have found themselves in............Now think about what they need to overcome their difficulties............strength and courage............tolerance of their own inevitable distress............sympathy and empathy for their own situation............support for themselves as opposed to judgement and self-criticism.

If you find it difficult to feel compassion for them that is OK............ maybe focus on your own behaviour towards the individual instead and your good intentions towards them............maybe the compassionate feelings will come later.

Focus your compassionate mind and all its key qualities on that person for a few minutes.

When you are ready, gently bring an end to the exercise and become more aware of your physical environment.

Reflection on Exercise 32

While some people find this exercise extremely easy, others find it incredibly difficult. For example, some people find that despite feeling an almost total lack of compassion for themselves, and a high level of self-criticism, they can very easily be compassionate towards others in a similar position. Although compassion for others is important, it can be problematic if we do not have equal compassion for ourselves too.

Others find this exercise extremely difficult because they see themselves in the person they are imagining, and this may lead to them becoming critical/undermining of their own situation and struggles. Their self-critic may become very negative towards the subject of this exercise. Whatever the issue is, people can find it difficult to be around others who remind them of their own situation, and can find themselves being inadvertently hostile towards fellow sufferers. If this is the case for you, take some reassurance from the fact that it is very common. It does, however, mean that you may need to gently nurture this capacity within yourself, attempting to build it up just as you are attempting to build your self-confidence. Here are some ideas for strategies that others with the same problem have found helpful:

- Engage in the exercise again, and whenever you become mindful of being critical towards the subject, bring your attention back to a mindfulness exercise, soothing breathing rhythm or place of contentment. Once you have done this, engage with your compassionate mind and return to the exercise.

- Focus the exercise on an individual who is a little *less* lacking in self-confidence, maybe focusing on someone who shows a lack of self-confidence in one area of their life but is confident in other areas.

- Engage in the exercise while focusing compassion on a timid animal. This may seem odd but we are attempting to 'train your brain' ultimately towards developing self-compassion for your own struggles. It does not matter where you start, only where you end up.

Exercise 33: Turning compassion inwards

In preparation for this exercise, bring to mind a childhood situation when you struggled with something. It could be with your homework, or in a particular class; it could be in a specific social situation or with a particular sport. As with the previous exercises, try not to concentrate on a situation that was charged with very strong emotions as this may be counter-productive. Instead start with something that is neither too charged with emotion nor devoid of it, but somewhere in the middle.

Find a place where you can be for 10–15 minutes that is, as far as possible, free from distractions. Sit in a relaxed, open posture that has *strength* or *alertness* in it. Close your eyes or settle your gaze on a low fixed point.

Settle your mind and body, maybe through your soothing breathing rhythm, maybe your place of contentment.

Now open up to your compassionate mind, and all the sensory experiences this brings with it............maybe assuming the role of a deeply compassionate person............maybe evoking compassion through a memory............maybe assuming your ideal compassionate self.

Gently bring to mind a situation when, as a child, you found yourself struggling............For a moment observe yourself............With your compassionate mind, experience compassion for yourself as that child............care for well-being............sympathy and empathy............ability to tolerate and contain the distress............sensitivity and attention to the distress............non-judgement............doing all of this in the context of warmth.

When you are ready, gently bring the exercise to an end and become more aware of your physical environment.

Reflection on Exercise 33

This exercise can prove difficult as it may evoke troubling memories, emotions, thoughts and feelings. This is why you are asked to do this exercise in relation to a childhood situation. Although they can often be associated with sadness, childhood memories tend to be less weighted with self-criticism and are consequently easier to view with compassion.

Developing compassion towards one aspect of yourself, at one time in your life, can be a stepping stone to becoming more self-compassionate generally.

Exercise 34: Compassion for your own journey and situation

In this exercise you will return to one you have previously undertaken and see how you view it in light of the new knowledge you have acquired in this chapter. Hopefully you will bring to it a deeper understanding and emotional connectedness to your current situation and journey.

In preparation, familiarize yourself once more with the formulation you drew out in Chapter 4. This was the diagrammatic representation of the factors leading up to your current situation, and the things that seem to maintain it. It specifically looked at the origins of your lack of self-confidence and what has prevented you from building it.

Now, finding a place where you can be for 10–15 minutes that is, as far as possible, free from distractions, sit in a relaxed, open posture that has *strength* or *alertness* in it. Close your eyes or settle your gaze on a low fixed point. Settle your mind and body, maybe through your soothing breathing rhythm, maybe your 'place of contentment' exercise.

Awaken your compassionate mind, and all the sensory experiences this brings with it...........maybe assuming the role of a deeply compassionate person...........maybe evoking compassion through a memory...........maybe assuming the ideal compassionate self.

Reminding yourself of the compassionate mind's attributes........... experience a pure sense of care for well-being...........sympathy...........empathy...........tolerance of distress...........sensitivity and non-judgement...........Feel the wisdom of your compassionate mind...........the warmth...........the strength and courage........... feel the commitment to resolve difficulties and move towards well-being...........feel these qualities in both your mind and your body.

Once you have evoked a sense of compassion, no matter how small or however fleeting, open your eyes and slowly, gently and warmly read through your formulation...........Take time to reflect on the words and their meaning in turn...........staying with each point or sentence until you feel as though you connect with what is written.

Take as much time as you need to read through, reflect and emotionally absorb what you have written – and, most importantly, what you have experienced or continue to experience.

When you feel you are ready, gently end the exercise by becoming more aware of your physical environment.

Reflection on Exercise 34

The purpose of this exercise is to turn your formulation into a more emotional experience. Again, for some this can be done relatively easily, while for others it can be more difficult.

If you are able to develop compassion for past and present circumstances, it is likely that the exercise will have been associated with some degree of emotion. For some that emotion can be extremely strong, for others less so. Maybe you found that you were able to connect emotionally with only some aspects of what you had written, or maybe with the formulation as a whole.

Whether you felt more emotion this time or not, it may be useful to return to this exercise and try it again. Some people find it helpful to rewrite their formulation after completing this exercise, this time using more compassionate language or else adding to it. We will return to your formulation once more and use it in the compassionate letter writing exercise later in this book, but for the time being it may be useful to reflect upon the difference that switching to a compassionate mindset makes.

Quote of Note:

'When there is no enemy within, the enemies outside cannot hurt you'

– African proverb

Exercise 35: Developing your compassionate coach

The previous exercise aimed to develop or enhance compassion for your own experiences and current situation. Here we will look at how to develop your *compassionate coach*, which will help you generate a compassionate mindset. Your *compassionate coach* won't be critical or hostile, forever pointing out what you have done wrong and undermining you.

Instead, similar to the supportive teacher in Chapter 3, your *compassion-ate coach* will work to build your self-confidence in a more helpful and meaningful way. Sometimes it may help you be more understanding of and kinder towards yourself. At other times it may *coach* you in how to approach external factors, giving you the strength to negotiate the important situations you face, and, perhaps more importantly, helping you feel more confident in everyday life too.

As with other imagery exercises, some people develop very detailed mental images of their coach that have the quality of a cartoon or maybe a photograph. Others develop merely a hazy impression of their compassionate coach. It doesn't matter which kind you develop, the most important thing is the qualities your coach possesses, how they coach you and how you feel in their presence.

Now, finding a place where you can be for 5–10 minutes that is, as far as possible, free from distractions, sit in a relaxed, open posture that has *strength* or *alertness* in it. Close your eyes or settle your gaze on a low fixed point.

Awakening your compassionate mind, and all the sensory experiences this brings with it............maybe assuming the role of a deeply compassionate person............maybe evoking compassion through a memory............ maybe assuming the ideal compassionate self............Now imagine an ideal compassionate coach............Someone who has your best interests at heart............someone who concentrates purely on your well-being.

What kind of qualities would they have?............Imagine them being sympathetic to your difficulties............Imagine that they always know what you need............sometimes offering gentle encouragement............ sometimes motivating you............other times simply being alongside you in difficult situations............Imagine them being tolerant of all the emotions you feel and show............sensitive and non-judgemental.

Imagine how it feels to be in the presence of their infinite wisdom............ their warmth............their strength and courage............feel their commitment to resolving any difficulties you have and to building your self-confidence.

Spend a short time imagining your compassionate coach............their qualities of compassion............the sensory experience as you receive it ....Imagine being in their presence and how that feels in your mind and in your body.

Whenever you feel ready, finish the exercise and gently become aware of your physical environment.

The compassionate coach

Your compassionate coach does not replace the need to have *real* people around you and to build your self-confidence in relation to them. However, such imagery does have many advantages:

- A *compassionate coach* can be especially useful to those who do not have supportive people around them.
- They are always available, unlike human beings who aren't *'hung at back o' t'door'*. (In the Yorkshire saying!)
- They can help the way we relate to ourselves and the way we relate to others, thus making it more likely that we will develop meaningful 'real' relationships in the future.
- A compassionate coach can be a helpful bridge for those who find it difficult to be compassionate towards themselves.
- They can be used to help prepare us for other parts of this approach, such as 'taking action' and looking at our thoughts, which we will do later in this book.
- They can help us be more *mindful* and less *reactive*.

Reflections on Exercise 35

For those who develop clear visual images of their coach, these can range from someone similar to a sports coach, an older woman or man, a teacher, right through to a tree, a fairy, an angel or even a particular place.

Some find that the image that most easily comes to mind is that of someone they once knew or know now. But where possible it is helpful to avoid 'real people', alive or dead, for two reasons. First, human beings are never 'perfect' and what you are trying to create here is an 'ideal' compassionate coach. Secondly, it is likely that real people will trigger a range of emotions within us, and this may make it difficult for us to focus on the exercise or indeed on pure compassion. If this is the case for you it may be helpful to blend the individual with something else, so as to give them a non-human dimension that allows them to be removed in your mind from anything or anyone else.

Following on from this, you may also find that the term 'coach' isn't the right one for you. Ken Goss, in his book *The Compassionate Mind Approach to Beating Overeating*, uses the idea of an 'ideal compassionate companion', while in her work with those who have experienced trauma, Deborah Lee uses the term 'perfect nurturer'. Maybe 'compassionate teacher' or 'compassionate guide' would work better for you. Interestingly, some people find that one image is helpful in a particular situation while another may be more helpful in a different scenario. Some people like to have a mixture of male and female images. Who knows? Play around with the ones that help you most, and you may end up with a whole gang around you! Just concentrate on finding what works best for you.

The Cherokee story: the wolves within

A Native American elder was teaching his grandchildren about life. He said to them, 'A fight occurs within me ... it is a terrible fight between two wolves. One wolf represents fear, anger, envy, sorrow, regret, greed, arrogance, self-pity, resentment, inferiority, lies, false pride, superiority and ego. The other stands for joy, peace, love, hope, sharing, serenity, humility, kindness, benevolence, friendship, empathy, generosity, truth, compassion and faith. This same fight is going on inside you, and inside every other person too,' he added. The grandchildren thought about this for a minute and then one child asked his grandfather, 'Which wolf will win?' The old Cherokee paused for a moment and then warmly replied, 'The one you feed'.

Conclusions

Once developed, your compassionate mind acts as a foundation stone on which to build your self-confidence. It can 'tone down' your threat system and equip you with the necessary attributes, skills and qualities to stand tall and face life's difficulties.

Just as you were previously encouraged to practise mindfulness wherever and whenever it felt right for you, attempt to bring the exercises from this chapter into your everyday life also. This may involve setting aside some time each day to practise them. Later on, you may find that you set aside specific times less frequently but can instead incorporate these practices easily into your regular life, engaging in them, for instance, whenever you have a hot drink, while out on a walk or when watering the plants.

10 Using Compassionate Thinking in Response to Our Own Undermining

We have already seen how our minds can become a playground for undermining thoughts, images and views of ourselves. These are frequently accompanied by difficult emotions, a range of physical sensations, and certain accompanying behaviours. In this chapter we will look at ways of addressing our tendency to undermine ourselves, by using compassionate thinking.

Compassionate thinking, in relation to self-confidence, involves warmly understanding ourselves: both the factors that have influenced us in the past, and those that influence us now in our moment-to-moment living. It involves being empathic to the difficulties we may have, and can help us develop the strength and courage to address them.

This chapter will focus on:

• Understanding our thinking and the views we may hold

• Noticing thoughts and images that occur in our mind

• Generating compassionate alternative thoughts and images – evaluating thoughts that can undermine us, from the perspective of both the rational and the compassionate mind

• Using two chairs to strengthen your compassionate mind

Understanding Our Thinking and the Views We May Hold

We can have a number of different things running through our minds at any one time. Sometimes these thoughts and images relate to general everyday things, but if we struggle with self-confidence it is likely that many of our thoughts and images relate to ruminations about things that *have* happened and worries about things that *may* happen. Events in our everyday life can also trigger thoughts about the kind of person we believe we are, as well as how we view others and the world in general.

As if this weren't enough, we can have an additional layer of thoughts about the thoughts themselves. In other words, we often tell ourselves off for the way that we think, concluding 'there's something wrong with me', 'If only I could think more positively', or 'I must be weird to think like this'.

In preparation for the exercises later in this chapter we will reflect on why we, as human beings, think in certain ways and how our views develop. We will also look at why it may take time to change these patterns of thinking. We will then discuss how we can recruit our *new brain* to assist us in our efforts.

Our amazing brain capacity can be a double-edged sword

Let's remind ourselves of the extent of the brain's development. As human beings we have the capacity for complex thought *and* thoughts about thoughts (often referred to as *metacognition*). This allows us to run a commentary on our everyday lives, in the moment, as events unfold. We can reflect on past events and predict future ones by way of a narrative or images. All of this has been hugely important for the survival of our species. Our brains have evolved in ways that help us see the links between things, understand other people's behaviour and motivations, prepare us for predicted events in the future, work out risk factors associated with past events, and allow us to shift into the world of our imagination.

However, because our brains also have a 'better safe than sorry' factory setting (designed to protect us) this can leave us more likely to focus on the things we find difficult (be they in the past, present or future) and on trying to work them out. This can generate difficult emotions in us, as well as physical sensations and, of course, accompanying thoughts and images. A key point to remember is that all of this happens through *no fault of our own*, but is the product of our brain and biology plus the life experiences we have had.

Change Occurs Step by Step

At times, we can readily change our opinions and thoughts about things. For example, you might already have experienced a 'penny drop moment' when reading something in this book, which has changed your views and thoughts almost immediately.

However, at other times, changing the way we think, or how we view ourselves, is a more gradual process. Three factors influence this. Firstly, how our brains process information, secondly how much time we have spent thinking in a certain way and therefore 'training our brain', and thirdly how long it takes for us to learn something new.

How our brains process information

Research has shown that in order to help us navigate the complex world we live in, and the constant barrage of information around us, over time the brain has developed a way of drawing snap conclusions and making instantaneous predictions. Its main focus is reserved for 'more important things'. We experience conclusions and predictions in the form of the *beliefs* and *assumptions* and they apply to our physical surroundings and the people within them as well as to our own physical attributes and the type of person we are. The brain assumes all such beliefs and assumptions to be true. It will readily accept things that confirm its views, but can often reject or modify information that is inconsistent with these. Susan's story will help illustrate this.

Susan's story

Susan had grown up being told that she was *'useless'* and was treated that way by her family. Her mother and father and even her younger siblings would automatically do everything for her, assuming that she was *'unable'* to help herself, and would poke fun at her whenever the family got together. She quickly learnt constantly to defer to others and accepted her own *'uselessness'* as a fact. As an adult, whenever she came across situations that confirmed this view, she readily accepted them as further proof or evidence that she was, indeed, useless. Susan did not recognize her own achievements or personal strengths, and even when she did receive evidence of them, when things went well for her she would quickly dismiss this by saying it was 'down to luck', someone was just trying to be nice to her or, more worryingly, people were trying to manipulate her for their own ends. For example, despite getting a job that she enjoyed upon leaving school, and slowly working her way up into management, Susan could not see that this in any way reflected her own skills or attributes. She would state that she 'was in the right place at the right time', and even wondered whether her mother or father had orchestrated things for her. Upon receiving promotion, she thought, 'There's only me available to do the job. If there was any competition they wouldn't have promoted me.'

From Susan's example we can see how our brains sometimes fix us in a seemingly never-ending pattern that further reinforces the negative way we view ourselves. Changing this takes time and effort.

The time we have spent 'training our brain' in a particular way of thinking

If you have been viewing yourself in a certain way all your life you will have been engaging in this way of thinking for hundreds of thousands of hours. When I consciously started to work on my own self-confidence I was thirty-four. This meant that I had already been thinking, behaving, and feeling in a particular way about myself for approximately 297,024 hours! Look at the calculation below to work out how many hours you have spent 'training your brain' so far.

Age	Hours
20	175,200
30	262,800
40	350,400
50	438,000
60	525,600
70	613,200
80	700,800
90	788,400

Of course, you are not awake for all of this time, and the negative view you have of yourself may only have begun when you were in your teens or early twenties, but it is worthwhile working out just how many hours you may have spent thinking of yourself in a particular way. It is usually a shocking total, and can help us to understand why it sometimes takes us a great deal of time and effort to make fundamental changes in ourselves.

How long it takes to learn new skills

On average, those who pass their driving tests have received 47 hours of private instruction and have supplemented this with 20 hours of private practice. Achieving any new skill takes time and effort, which is why we often refer to Compassion Focused Therapy and the compassionate mind approach as 'physiotherapy for the brain'. We build up to changing things, step by step.

The exercises in this book can actually produce long-term changes in the brain, but such brain 'pathways' can be difficult to develop and use at first, just as you may find it difficult to find a path through the woods that has only been walked a few times before. Other pathways, such as self-critical ones, can be easier to find – but we know what happens if we only follow those. The action we most need to take is to repeatedly and purposefully walk the new pathways, which will in time make them easier to find and follow. The aim is to make these more attractive to us than the old ones, until all of a sudden we find that we no longer have to make a conscious effort to switch to them. Following the path of change becomes automatic for us.

How We Can Recruit Our New Brain to Assist Us in Our Efforts

The good news is that our *new brain* has the capacity to reason with our old one and, where appropriate, calm it down or soothe it. More specifically, we can use our new brain to allow us to step back from our own unruly mind and gain a better perspective on what is happening. We can re-evaluate situations using our *new brain*, often leading to different responses, different ways of viewing things and different emotions.

Noticing thoughts and images that occur in our mind

Some people find that they are already very aware of the thoughts and images that occupy their mind and undermine their self-confidence. If this is the case for you, you may choose to skip the next two exercises, proceeding straight to Exercise 38. However, if at the moment you find it difficult to identify or describe such thoughts and images, this section will help you.

The purpose of these exercises is two fold. Firstly, by becoming more aware of what is running through our minds we can, at times, become more objective, as opposed to just accepting our thoughts as facts. In other words, increased self-awareness can change our relationship with our own thoughts. Secondly, an awareness of the thoughts and images that undermine our self-confidence can give us new material to explore later.

Exercise 36: Recognizing thoughts and images that have occupied your mind

This exercise will ask you to reflect on three areas.

1. First, think back to the exercises in Chapters 7, 8 and 9. These involved mindfulness, further preparation for compassion and developing the compassionate mind. During these exercises, were you aware of any thoughts or images (recurring or not) that popped into your mind and knocked your self-confidence? These may have related to events in the past, present or future. If you are aware of any, make a note of them in your notebook or journal.

2. Now review all the notes you have been taking while working your way through this book. Can you identify any self-undermining thoughts and/or images that may have prevented you from building your self-confidence? If you do, circle them or write them out separately.

3. Finally, thinking back over the last week or month, were there any particular times when you felt as though your self-confidence had been knocked? If there were, bring to mind a situation you feel comfortable with returning to.[18] Imagine yourself back in that situation again for just a few moments. Close your eyes to help you reconnect with the experience. Now ask yourself the questions found in the box on page 158 and make some notes.

    Once you feel you have explored the situation sufficiently, engage in your soothing rhythm breathing or your preferred imagery exercise to access your soothing system.

---

[18]   Returning your mind to a specific situation is difficult, but if you still wish to review it, it may help to use your soothing rhythm breathing, place of contentment or compassion exercises at set intervals during the course of the exercise.

Questions to guide exploration of your thoughts and images

What was I thinking of in general in that situation?

What was the anxious part of my brain thinking . . .

. . . about thoughts and images that relate to me, to other people or the world in general?

What was the sad part of my brain thinking . . .

. . . about thoughts and images that relate to me, to other people or the world in general?

What was the angry part of my brain thinking . . .

. . . about thoughts and images that relate to me, to other people or the world in general?

What was the envious part of my brain thinking . . .

. . . about thoughts and images that relate to me, to other people or the world in general?

What do I fear most about this situation?

Have you noticed any self-critical or undermining thoughts or images going through your mind during this exercise?

Are there any rules you are aware of that, in this situation, you are applying to yourself, to other people or the world in general?

Susan's example illustrates how she worked through the three elements of this exercise. As you can see, the prompts she used helped her identify a whole range of different thoughts and emotions, all generated from the same situation.

Susan's notes from Exercise 36:

Thoughts and images I can now recognize that undermine my self-confidence

1.   In relation to exercises in chapters 7–9:

     I can't focus my mind, I'm useless at this

     I don't deserve to feel compassionate about myself

     Change isn't happening fast enough

2.   From my journal:

     Images of my mum wagging her finger at me

     I'm pathetic

     I've got to get on and change things because I am wasting my life

     I'll never get the hang of this

3.   In relation to my boss recently criticizing my work:

     I'm rubbish . . . useless

     I'm going to be found out as someone who can't do their job

     I'm never going to feel any different

     Doesn't she realize I am trying my hardest

     It's not fair. Paula did something very similar and she gets away with everything

     I'm going to lose this job

     I'll never achieve anything

     There's no point in trying so hard at work because my best isn't good enough

---

Exercise 37: Noticing thoughts and images as they occur in your mind

In order to recognize thoughts and images that are occupying your mind and undermining your self-confidence, this exercise will ask you to reflect in two different ways.

1.   Rather than reflecting on past events, diary entries and practices, start to make notes relating to your practice of mindfulness or compassionate imagery in difficult situations *over the coming week*. After completing each exercise jot down in your notebook or journal any undermining thoughts and images that your mind has wandered to.

2.   Over the week ahead identify and explore situations in which your self-confidence has been knocked *as they occur* and warmly bring your attention to whatever thoughts and images are occupying your mind at the time. If you find this difficult, look out for variations in your emotions, physical sensations or certain behaviours as 'markers' or prompts. For example, some people find that the first thing they notice is a sense of dread or anxiety, maybe anger. Others notice physical sensations such as a faster heart-rate, sweating, a dry mouth, tension or a sense of heaviness. Some people may notice that they feel dirty or contaminated and have the urge to wash. Others note that they crave food, alcohol or a cigarette when they know they don't *need* it, or may start to pick at their skin or scratch.

All of these behaviours should be viewed as prompts, reminding us to ask ourselves: 'What is running through my mind right now?' Engaging with your soothing rhythm breathing at such times can help you 'warmly observe'. You can then ask yourself similar questions to those outlined in the previous box, replacing 'what was' with 'what is' and so forth. It may be helpful to have the questions written down in your notebook or journal, and to have this ready for use when a difficult situation arises.

Reflection on Exercises 36 and 37

As you go through these exercises it can be tempting to (and almost impossible not to) try and work out what happened in light of what you are feeling now. If this is the case for you, just acknowledge that it is a common tendency to get caught up in all manner of 'workings out' and then return to becoming aware of thoughts and images with curiosity.

Whether you are reflecting on a difficult situation or in the middle of one, your soothing rhythm breathing can bring your soothing system 'on-line' and allow you space and time to think things through. That said, some people find that this is so effective it 'turns off' their thoughts and/ or prevents them from being able to access them. Use the practice in the manner that is most helpful to you.

Although there is an emphasis placed on noticing thoughts and images associated with specific situations, many people find that their thoughts and images are not limited to a particular situation currently in progress. Thoughts and images from the past, as well as thoughts and predicted images of the future, may also occur.

For example, in social situations David had thoughts such as 'They think I am boring' or 'I just can't gel with people', and this led to others like 'I'm never going to meet a partner', and mental images of himself ten years older, still living in a flat on his own.

Valerie found that whenever she felt anxious in social situations, she not only had thoughts such as 'I look really anxious' and 'People are noticing I am anxious and are judging me', she also had a visual image of herself looking red and flustered together with one of herself in the playground at school, being taunted by other children.

Whether the thoughts and images that you notice are limited to the present situation, or also include the past, the future or both, the key is just to notice this and bring such thoughts into your awareness.

More on 'physiotherapy for the brain'

If we want to develop our biceps, simply raising our arms up and down from the elbow is unlikely to have the desired effect. Neither would it be a good idea to try and lift too big a weight straight away. Although such techniques *can* have *some* effect, we actually have to work against a comfortable amount of resistance in order to make the changes we need to make sensibly and efficiently.

This is also true for the work you are embarking on now. If the exercises were easy it would indicate that this is not where you necessarily need to be directing your efforts. If, on the other hand, certain exercises seem too hard, and produced very high levels of emotion, this also is a less than effective use of your time and effort. You need to work at an intensity that produces the best results for you – that is achievable but not too easy. And whenever you feel over-stretched, use a mindfulness or soothing exercise for a period of time until the emotions subside, just as you would take a break at the gym.

Compassionate Alternative Thoughts and Images

Once you have begun to notice the thoughts and images that are occupying your mind and undermining your self-confidence, generating compassionate alternatives may help your 'new brain' to change this pattern for the better. Doing this can help us to stand back from a situation and, instead of jumping to conclusions, making assumptions and imposing rules, to take a more rounded and realistic viewpoint instead. This way, it is less likely we will be biased and emotionally controlled by the thoughts and images in our heads. In the following exercise we will be asking your new brain to respond to your old brain and, through this process, help you reach conclusions that reflect all of the brain's capacity rather than just one side of it.

A question of balance:

Understandably some people may wonder: 'What if my old brain was right?' 'What if people really *are* judging me negatively?' 'What if I *am* being considered for redundancy?' 'What if my partner *is* having an affair?'

Generating compassionate alternative thoughts isn't about overruling any instincts that you may have, but about allowing yourself to look at the broader picture and to draw a more considered conclusion. If you then conclude that your initial instincts were right, your *new brain* can help you deal with this. It can give you the strength and courage to cope with difficult things; it can help you face any pain and upset, and remind you of your own resilience; it can bring to mind other difficulties you have faced and coped with in the past; it can prepare you and coach you through the most trying situations.

By now you are probably more aware of the range of thoughts and images that run through your mind in different situations. We are going to look specifically at those that undermine your self-confidence.

To generate compassionate alternative thoughts and experience[19] their benefits the compassionate mind approach recommends the following 5 steps.

Step 1 involves writing down difficult thoughts and images that you are having or have become aware of, on a compassionate thoughts/images worksheet.

Step 2 involves engaging with the pragmatic part of your brain – the reporter rather than the interrogator – and using it to gain a more balanced perspective of the information at hand. It is not a matter of 'kidding

---

[19] The term 'experience' is used here to recognize that the aim of the exercise is to generate alternative thoughts but importantly also to *feel* the effect that having such thoughts has on us, therefore turning an intellectual exercise into an emotional one.

yourself' into new ways of thinking, but of drawing conclusions that are considered and balanced. The text box on page 163 is designed to help you with this.

Step 3 involves using your compassionate mindset to help generate a different, more compassionate perspective on your thoughts and images. This may be through use of the ideal compassionate self, the perfect nurturer or your compassionate coach – whichever you feel would be the most helpful to you. The questions found in the text box below are designed to help you with this.

Step 4 involves once again using your compassionate mind and, re-reading what you have written, allowing each new conclusion to have more emotional impact. As we discovered in Chapter 9, your compassionate mind has the ability to support you through difficult feelings and times. This can help turn something you *know* into something you *feel*.

Step 5 involves looking over what you have written and experienced and potentially finding ways to build further upon it. The following text box may assist you with this.

Questions to ask when reviewing your worksheet

Are the thoughts I have written helpful to me?

When I read out what I have written (be it in my head or out loud) is the tone of my voice warm, soothing and ultimately helpful?

Can I evoke a sense of warmth when I read through the alternatives generated?

Before you start, let's look at Harry's story and how he used this exercise.

Harry's story

Harry struggled with his self-confidence. This was largely due to difficulties he had had at school. Although naturally quite shy, Harry found himself in a group of very confident boys, all of whom came from quite affluent backgrounds. Harry's family, on the other hand, struggled to make ends meet. He wore his older brother's old clothes and was unable to attend many school trips and after-school clubs. At the age of 13 Harry's family moved a little bit further away from school. Subsequently, Harry did not have as many opportunities to see his friends and became more isolated. He felt angry that his friends did not make any effort to travel to see him, instead expecting him to come to them. Harry decided to broach the subject but instead of sorting things out it led to a big argument and his friendships with them were never the same again. Feeling low, Harry withdrew from his family, and feelings of inadequacy took over. He became anxious in a range of situations, especially in classes where his old friends were. Harry coped by constantly monitoring himself for signs that he might look anxious to others. He also found that he became extremely careful about what he said to people for fear that they would reject him. At the age of 15, when a boy his own age moved in next door and joined the school, life turned a corner. They got on well straight away, and in helping the 'new kid on the block' become familiar with the local area and school Harry found he was able to rebuild some of his self-confidence. However, the preceding two years had taken their toll and all of this left Harry with a tendency to feel anxious and inadequate.

As an adult Harry found that in a range of stressful situations his mind would become full of undermining thoughts. Although some were very specific to the situation he found himself in, he could identify key themes that recurred across various situations. As Step 1 Harry recorded these in the first column of his worksheet (see page 168). After noticing and recording his undermining thoughts and images, Harry then used the questions in the text box on page 167, to help him come up with rational alternatives. He recorded these in the second column of the worksheet (Step 2).

Step 3 involved Harry recruiting his compassionate mind to help him gain a more compassionate perspective on his situation. He chose to do this by first engaging in his soothing rhythm breathing. After a few minutes he then evoked the image of his ideal compassionate self and reminded himself of the key attributes and qualities of compassion, feeling them in his own mind and body. In this mindset, he examined each of his undermining thoughts and slowly responded to each situation compassionately. He used the questions in the text box on page 167 to help him respond compassionately to his own distressing thoughts.

For step 4 Harry chose to add each of his compassionate responses to the bottom of the worksheet. Alternatively he could have chosen to link them specifically to each of the points in the first column, embedding them within the worksheet. His additional thoughts and images are recorded below.

Harry's additional compassionate thoughts/images

Things are often difficult – life can be hard.

It is understandable that I feel as I do about things.

Some people do make judgements and there are often things I cannot control – this can be difficult.

Such things don't happen only to me.

I have had a difficult time and it is understandable that I still struggle with things.

Of course I want things to be better but it may be more helpful to support myself rather than undermine myself – retain the image of the compassionate versus the critical teacher, seeing myself walking towards the compassionate one and standing by her side.

I am building my self-confidence and it helps me to use my compassionate coach's strength and wisdom.

It helps to be understanding of my difficulties, yet to learn from setbacks and use them to help me move forward.

Questions to ask to help you generate alternative viewpoints

If I stand back from this situation, could there be another way of viewing it?

Is there any evidence that would not support the conclusions I have drawn?

If I wasn't experiencing strong emotions would I think any differently about the situation, about myself or about other people?

If I was looking back in a year from now would I view things in the same way?

If a friend was thinking in this way what would I say to them?

What would I want a friend to say to me?

What would............(someone who cared or cares about you) say?

Are there occasions in the past when I have thought this way but the conclusions I drew proved to be incorrect?

Even if I were correct are there things that I could say to myself that would be helpful?

Am I expecting unrealistic things of myself, other people or the situation?

What may be or might have been going on for the other person/people involved?

Is it more about other people or the situation than it is about me?

Harry's compassionate alternative thoughts and imagery worksheet

Undermining thoughts/images	Alternative thoughts/images
I'm going to mess up	I never totally screw up – there are many times that I can recall where things have gone well – on the whole I am doing OK. Just because something isn't 'perfect' it doesn't mean I have messed up. My anxiety and threat system is talking, that's what it does, it is unlikely to be right.
People are watching me and judging me negatively	Even if I do mess things up I will learn from this and grow. People judge me less than I think they do – it's just my anxiety talking when I am in the middle of an anxiety-provoking situation. Some people are willing me on to do well. I have had good feedback in the past – sometimes about me as a person or my work. In actual fact it's hard to like someone who is 'perfect' so I shouldn't try to be. Julie often looks anxious in meetings and I don't think any the worse of her – I actually think it's quite endearing. Tom always presents himself and his work really well but I know he struggles in other areas.
I'm a waste of space	I can't be that bad as I have managed to remain in this job for over twelve months. There are aspects of myself that I am happy with. I have some good friends who seem to want to spend time with me. I have a range of positive qualities, I am a good listener, I can have a laugh.
I'm going to be alone	No one can say for definite whether they are going to end up alone or not – all I can do is increase my chances of meeting someone and ensure I have some good friends around me.
Things always go wrong/images of key times when things have gone wrong	There are times when things have gone right – they are just difficult to access when I am feeling low or anxious. I have been successful in a couple of interviews. I managed to rent a good flat. I have had some good nights out, I have some good friendships and enjoy a number of things.
Why do I do this to myself all the time – I am so annoying	I continue to put myself up for things because I want things to be better – I want to grow. We all have to start somewhere and I cannot expect never to make mistakes. It may be helpful to think of myself as being 'in training' – by 'putting myself out there', be it in work or in relationships, I am being courageous but there will be times when I am disappointed.

Harry had a short break and then, in the penultimate step of this exercise (Step 4), he once again evoked a compassionate mindset. He engaged in his soothing rhythm breathing and then brought to mind his compassionate coach. In this frame of mind Harry then *slowly* read through all the alternative compassionate thoughts and images, allowing time for each of them to resonate with him. This helped the alternatives have more impact and reduced his 'old brain's' capacity to dismiss them.

Finally, Harry asked himself the questions in the box on page 167. He reflected that when he re-read his letter he automatically did so in a warm and soothing tone, and he experienced the reflections as truly helpful to him.

In time he found that repeated use of this exercise made it easier for him to readily access such thoughts *and* associated feelings, not only while carrying out exercises to improve his self-confidence but also when he actually found himself in difficult situations.

Of course, this is a very comprehensive example, designed to show an across-the-board approach to one person's problems. You personally may find it easier to start off by just picking one undermining thought or image at a time and working through it in isolation, rather than attempting to work through all of your problems at once.

Generating Compassionate Alternative Thoughts

Instead of habitually focusing on the thoughts and images that undermine your self-confidence, the following exercise will help you generate compassionate thoughts instead. Remember, the emphasis is on finding something that works for you. Don't worry too much about getting the exercise 'right', or being neat or concise. Throw yourself into it and explore what is in your mind and what alternatives you can come up with.

Exercise 38 : Giving your new and compassionate brain a voice

Remember the steps:

1. Notice and record any difficult thoughts and images.

2. Generate alternative thoughts and images.

3. Use a compassionate mind exercise to generate further alternatives.

4. While in your compassionate mindset, slowly read through the alternative thoughts and images you have come up with, allowing time for them to sink in and have an emotional impact on you.

5. Review what you have written.

Don't forget to use the questions listed in the text boxes previously to help you at each stage.

Reflection on Exercise 38

Some people find that they can come up with alternative thoughts and images, be they pragmatic or compassionate, without the need to write things down – and at times this is the only option. For example, it would be hard to write things down while driving, in the middle of a meeting or on a night out. However, more often than not, committing our thoughts to paper can help to focus our mind. While engaged in writing, people often find that they can keep their emotions in check and concentrate instead on working out the problem confronting them. I find that it's a bit like mental arithmetic – if I try to work things out in my mind, I get lost in all the ramifications. I also become easily distracted by what is going on around me. However, if I write things down, it's much easier for me to keep track of every aspect of the problem.

Step 5 of the process helps to highlight the things it may be beneficial for you to consider further. If you find, for example, that you experience doubts about certain alternative thoughts or images, evoke your compassionate mind once more and investigate matters further. Are there other

Worksheet 7 : My own compassionate alternative thoughts and images

Undermining thoughts/images	Compassionate alternative thoughts/images

things that you are telling yourself that may account for your feelings of doubt? Does the alternative perhaps arouse strong emotional responses in you? Is the critical part of yourself stepping in and undermining things for you again? Noticing sticking points can be really important as this will guide you towards areas that still need to be addressed before you can build your self-confidence further.

Finally, many people find it helpful to write down key 'alternative' compassionate thoughts on the front or back cover of their notebook or on postcards which they keep readily accessible. Brief statements that are personally significant, such as 'It is understandable that sometimes I struggle', may suffice. Others may prefer to write more comprehensive statements (or a combination of the two), such as, 'I have been through a lot . . . it takes time to build self-confidence. Each day I will nurture myself and use my courage to grow. When I have setbacks I will be both kind and encouraging to myself. I will then reflect and take a further step tomorrow.' Don't forget to use your soothing rhythm breathing and to evoke a compassionate mindset before reading them, in order to make them sink in.

Chair Work

Using two chairs to strengthen your compassionate mind

Having paid attention to the undermining or self-critical thoughts that run through our minds, and then generated compassionate alternatives, we will now see if a different use of the imagery work covered in Chapters 7 to 9 can be of further help in addressing our self-undermining.

Chair work is used in a number of ways in psychological therapy. In this instance, you will use it to evoke different aspects of yourself, namely the part of you that may be struggling as well as your compassionate mindset – this may be the ideal compassionate self, the perfect nurturer or your compassionate coach or teacher.

In Chapter 9 we looked at how particular smells, textures, music or pictures can help you to switch on your compassionate mindset. If you found this of help to you previously it may be beneficial to use these prompts again during this exercise.

Because people prefer to use different imagery to evoke a compassionate mindset, in this exercise we will refer to the 'compassionate role', be it the ideal compassionate self, the perfect nurturer or the compassionate coach/teacher.

Exercise 39: Two chairs

Begin by bringing to mind a situation where you have struggled, a time that evoked an emotional response in you. This may be a situation you have looked at in a previous exercise or one that you have written down in your notebook or journal. It will be something you are happy to work on now but which has previously made you feel anxious, low or angry, and has knocked your self-confidence.

Now place two chairs so that they are facing each other, not straight on but at a slight angle, maybe as you would arrange the chairs if a friend were visiting.

Now, sitting in one of the chairs, assume the role of the part of you that is struggling. Allow yourself to express your worries, concerns and frustrations out loud. It may feel quite uncomfortable or unnatural doing this at first. Because the exercise is focusing on your thoughts, try to stay with these rather than getting too deep into the associated emotions. Strong emotions can turn off the speech centres of the brain (this may be the origin of the phrase 'lost for words') and it is important that we get a conversation going here. Take time to voice everything that is troubling you.

Once you feel you have described the situation out loud, stand up and walk around for a while or sit quietly in a completely different chair. Practise your soothing rhythm breathing. When you are ready, sit down in the second chair. Assume your compassionate posture, with your spine strong but your body relaxed. Bring to mind the compassionate role that works best for you and experience the warmth that this evokes. As you engage your compassionate mind, imagine sitting in the presence of the part of you that is struggling; you may find that your facial expression softens. Remind yourself of the attributes and qualities of the compassionate role: tolerant of distress, warm and wise, non-judgemental, and possessing great courage. Experience these qualities, in your mind and in your body, for a few moments.

Now, with warmth in your voice and in your heart, speak to the part of you that is struggling. Maybe acknowledge that you are experiencing difficulties and that life is hard for you. Acknowledge the fact that a whole range of factors means you have found yourself in this difficult situation, and it is not your fault but a product of your biology and experiences. This might make you feel uncomfortable. If you find this to be the case just allow yourself time to settle, maybe again engaging in your soothing rhythm breathing. When you are ready, assume the role once more – just as an actor steps into the skin of someone they are attempting to portray.

Speaking out loud, address the struggling part of yourself. It may help to point out that many people struggle similarly and you are not alone in this. And perhaps remind yourself of the other times when you have overcome setbacks and grown from them.

When you feel as though the compassionate role you have inhabited has voiced all it wishes to share, stand up once again. After spending a little time in your soothing rhythm breathing, return to the first chair. Settle yourself for a moment. Now imagine yourself back into the first role, sitting in the presence of your compassionate self and hearing what they have to say, feeling their warmth towards you. Sit still and experience this sensation for a while.

Only when you feel that you have got the most you can from this exercise, and while keeping hold of the emotions it evoked in you, pick up your notebook or journal and jot down some reminders for yourself. Ask questions such as: what did the compassionate self say or want me to know? How did they perceive me, this situation, and others like it?

Once you feel you have recorded all the important points, stand up and walk around for a while. If this is difficult, you may choose to sit in a different chair altogether. Engage with your soothing rhythm breathing. When you are ready, sit down in the compassionate chair once more. Is there anything else you should add to your summary, other things you would like to say to the part of you that is struggling?

Finally, slowly read through the points that you have recorded. Allow yourself the time to experience the words and feel them emotionally.

Reflection on Exercise 39

When faced with this exercise, some people find a number of reasons not to do it. They fear they will find it uncomfortable and, understandably, want to avoid this. But my advice to them is: 'What have you got to lose?' You don't need to do this in the presence of others, you can do it in the privacy of your own home. And time and time again, people go on to report that, despite their initial reservations, having given it a go, they found it to be one of the most powerful exercises they tried.

Some report finding no reason to speak while in the compassionate role. Others tell me that they direct warmth or colours towards the self that is struggling, or else gentle waves of soothing energy. Having returned to the original chair they then find that this has helped. Some people seem to need a different way of viewing their situation before they can bring about an emotional change in themselves, whereas others find that they can experience such change without the need for this sort of role-playing. Of course, as ever, the key is finding something that works for you. However, I would always suggest *trying* to give the compassionate role a voice because it can be very effective.

Conclusions

It is apparent that the thoughts and images that occupy our minds can play a key role in undermining self-confidence. They can also help us to build it when combined with a compassionate frame of mind. In the next chapter we will look at compassionate letter writing as a means of further building self-confidence.

11 Compassionate Letter Writing

In this chapter you will learn how to use compassionate letter writing as a means of further exploring your own capacity for inner support and self-compassion. Such letters can also help you generate new ways of thinking and, at times, ideas about things it may be helpful for you to address. This in turn can help to build self-confidence.

After reading the guidelines below, you will be asked to write three specific letters. These will be:

1. a compassionate letter specifically focused on building your self-confidence;

2. a compassionate letter *from* the compassionate role *to* yourself;

3. a compassionate letter focusing on your own compassionate alternative thoughts and images worksheet (page 171).

Guidelines for Compassionate Letter Writing

Take time to experience what you are writing

During this exercise you will be asked to engage both the intellectual *and* the emotional part of your brain, so take your time and allow yourself to *feel* each sentence, phrase or word you use.

Take a break whenever it is helpful

Some people find it difficult to concentrate on letter writing and they become frustrated by this. Others find that focusing their efforts on certain things can evoke strong physical sensations: for example, a sense of numbness or difficult emotions such as sorrow, anger or anxiety. Although at times it is helpful to stay with these difficult experiences, at others it may be preferable to take a break. At such times it may help to evoke your compassionate mind via one of the imagery exercises or else by using your soothing rhythm breathing. It may also help to get up and move around for a time. Then, when you are ready, return to the exercise once more.

Alternatively it may help to make this the focus of your letter, or a subsequent one. You could write: 'As I sit here and write this letter it is understandable that I feel strong emotions because...........' Or, from a different perspective you may write: 'I am sorry that writing this letter is painful for you and evokes difficult emotions............I can understand why this would be...........you are courageous to embark on this work...........'

Your letter does not have to be perfect!

Don't worry about your handwriting, spelling or grammar. You may prefer to write in sentences and paragraphs. Alternatively, it may be helpful to build pauses into compassionate letters by the use of multiple full stops. For some people, this helps slow down the train of thought. For example, in part of the letter you may write something like:

...........it is not your fault...........stand tall...........breathe........... you are not alone...........others struggle...........connect.

Try not to let perfectionism and self-criticism cause you to over-think your letters. Remember, the aim of this exercise is to call upon self-compassion and inner support, not to achieve an A*.

My personal story about writing

At school I managed to develop a style of handwriting that I thought covered up my poor spelling and it worked for a while. By the time I got to secondary school my difficulties with word blindness and spelling were identified. This was a mixed blessing. Suddenly I had people to help me. Unfortunately, however, this was often done in a shaming way with a thick red marker pen and extra lessons before school every day. My poor handwriting was also picked up on, which, by now, was very difficult to correct. For both of these reasons, writing can be associated with difficult emotions for me but, when I do these exercises, it helps to reflect that my ideal compassionate self or compassionate coach is supportive of me and my efforts. They are not concerned about my handwriting, grammar or spelling. Instead they are concerned about the way I feel about myself.

Letters can be long or short

In some cases it only takes a few words to access inner support and self-compassion whereas for others more detail is required to get to the same place. Remember, it's not *how much* you write but *how it makes you feel*.

If it helps, build upon the work of others

There are a number of short examples of compassionate letters in this chapter and further examples can be found on the Compassionate Mind website (www.compassionatemind.co.uk). It may help you to look at some of these before starting this exercise. Guiding principles for compassionate letters can be found in the text box opposite.

Combine the practice with other things you have found useful

If you found that use of a particular smell, texture, picture or colour helped you to access your compassionate mind more readily, it may help to use such prompts during this exercise also.

Guiding principles for compassionate letters

Be sensitive to, and validate, the emotions you experience.

Convey understanding, acceptance and caring.

Validate the reasons why you may be struggling with certain things.

Recognize that we are a complex species and this means we often struggle.

Recognize that we are prone to self-criticism, and although your self-critic has your best intentions at heart, listening to it is not the best way to build self-confidence.

Remain non-judgemental.

Reflect on which of the three circles/emotional systems (see page 9) it would be helpful for you to work on at the moment.

Remind yourself that you are not on your own. Millions of other people struggle to build their self-confidence.

Recognize that life can be hard and sometimes other people can do things that hurt us.

Allow yourself to be moved by your own experiences rather than avoiding difficult situations.

Start when things are relatively easy

As with any of these exercises, it is best initially to embark on the process of compassionate letter writing when you are feeling relatively stable emotionally rather than when you are facing problems. As you become more familiar with the practice you can then use it at more difficult times.

Materials

All you need is your notebook, journal or a sheet of paper together with a pen or pencil. It may be helpful to have your notes and summary sheets from the previous exercises to hand to remind yourself of previous work you have done.

Exercise 40: Compassionate letter writing to build your self-confidence

As the aim of this book is to build your self-confidence we will start by writing a letter focused specifically on this. Because this is likely to be your first experience of compassionate letter writing a template is provided to guide you in this process.

We will then look at variations and adaptations for you to try. Hopefully some form of letter writing will eventually become an integral part of your ongoing self-confidence building. It may be of benefit to write down a few notes or reflections after you've carried out each exercise on your personal practice summary sheet (see page xxx) or in your notebook or journal.

While posture is an important factor in all exercises, in this one it is particularly important. You will be asked to adopt a self-confident posture. It is likely this will be similar, if not identical, to the posture you have found useful before – one with alertness and strength in it paired with warmth and openness. However, you may find that while writing there are slight differences. For example, it may be helpful to raise the chin slightly higher or imagine a core of strength running through your body. Alternatively, you may become aware of a sense of strength in the chest and experience an expansion in this area of the body.

Although this is not an essential element of all compassionate letters, in this exercise you will be encouraged to come up with ideas of what it may be helpful for you to do in relation to the building of your self-confidence. These ideas may then be used later in Chapter 12, which focuses on 'taking action'.

First, spend a little time re-familiarizing yourself with your compassionate formulation developed in Chapter 4. This diagram drew together your influences and experiences, concerns and fears, coping strategies you've been using and their unintended drawbacks.

Now, find a place that is, as far as possible, free from distractions. Somewhere you can be for an hour or so. If this seems too daunting, start by aiming to work on this exercise for just 10–15 minutes. Feel strength and alertness in your spine, with a relaxed and open posture.

If it is helpful to you, start by using your soothing rhythm breathing or 'place of contentment' exercise. Now use one of the imagery exercises outlined in Chapter 9 to evoke a compassionate mindset. Alternatively you can use one of the mindfulness practices described in Chapter 7 to create a sense of calm awareness, or else simply go straight into the exercise once your mind and body are settled.

Remind yourself of the compassionate attributes and qualities, such as warmth, non-judgement, empathy, wisdom and strength, feeling them in your mind and in your body. Feel a gentle smile on your face and adjust your posture to embody a sense of strength and self-confidence.

Now use the following template to guide you in your letter writing:

It is understandable that I have found it difficult to build my self-confidence because...
....
....
....

(Tip: include both past experiences and current circumstances – gently, with warmth, attempt to convey empathy and understanding in what you write.)

It is understandable that I have developed concerns and fears about...............
....
....
....
....

I have coped by..
....
....
....
....
....
....
....

But there have been unintended consequences and drawbacks, such as............
....
....
....
....
....
....
....

One of the unintended consequences is that my self-confidence has not developed. This is not my fault, but it is my responsibility to change my future.

(Tip: don't forget all the time you are writing your letter to retain your self-confident posture, with your chin up and a feeling of strength in the chest.)

Now I am committing myself to building my self-confidence but this will take time.

I recognize that I have the capacity for strength, courage, resilience and wisdom.

(Now imagine yourself being in the presence of your compassionate coach.)

My compassionate coach would remind me that.....................................
....
....
....
....
....
....

I have already taken a number of steps towards building my self-confidence. These include..

....

....

....

....

....

....

In the past, when I was struggling with difficult situations, it would have helped me if those around me had been more nurturing of my self-confidence and...

....

....

....

....

....

....

....

At the time it would have also helped me if I had done the following things to nurture myself and build my self-confidence..

....

....

....

....

....

....

....

With this in mind, it may be helpful for me now to...

....

....

....

....

....

....

(Tip: avoid shoulds, musts, etc. And, remember, the idea is to be encouraging and nurturing – therefore big goals can be broken down into small and manageable steps.)

If I had setbacks my compassionate coach would remind me that.................
....
....
....
....
....

The emotions they would direct my way would be...................................
....
....
....
....
....

When you feel you have written enough, put down your pen and centre yourself by doing one of the exercises you find helpful, such as your soothing rhythm breathing or visiting your place of contentment. Finally, slowly read through your letter, with a feeling of warmth and strength towards yourself, and allow the words to 'sink in'.

Andy's first compassionate letter

We first met Andy in Chapter 4. His difficulties with self-confidence had partly arisen from his family's overprotectiveness towards him during a long childhood illness, and in his teens and university days Andy had always felt socially isolated by his inability to be able to join his friends in sporting activities. Andy's experiences and feelings were charted in his formulation (see page 61). He later revisited it in order to write a compassionate letter to himself. As you can see, he has used the template above as a guide, but has focused on the bits of it that he found most relevant to him and changed some of the wording where appropriate.

It is understandable that I have found it difficult to build my self-confidence. I have been through a lot, with my physical health problems and having very confident siblings, to problems 'fitting in' with my sporty friends and using alcohol as a crutch. Given these things it would be unusual for someone not to be concerned about their physical health. I can understand why I often feel 'different' and therefore susceptible to feelings of social isolation. I have developed a sense of being an outsider because I have had these early experiences.

I have coped by doing all manner of things, from beating myself up to drinking and avoidance tactics. But these strategies have drawbacks that prevent me from building my self-confidence.

This is not my fault, but it is my responsibility to change my future. Now I am committing time and effort to building my self-confidence. I recognize that I have the capacity for strength, courage, resilience and wisdom, and my compassionate coach reminds me of these things. He also reminds me that he 'has my back' and, despite setbacks, with concerted efforts I can change things for the better.

I have already made a lot of progress. I have recognized this is an issue for me and bought this book. I have worked through the exercises so far, despite some difficulties and reservations.

I can't blame other people for my situation as I never let them know I was struggling. If I had, they could have encouraged and supported me. I am going to do this for myself but I am going to let certain people know what I am doing so I can gain their support.

I know I will have setbacks but at such times I will remind myself of the compassionate qualities and use the exercises in this book to practise self-compassion. I will grow and learn from each of my setbacks, recognizing that it is understandable for me to feel knocked by them, but looking at them as an opportunity to learn more about myself.

Reflection on Exercise 40

If you find that the concept of a compassionate coach is not helpful to you, you may prefer to use the ideal compassionate self, compassionate companion or teacher or perfect nurturer.

Although some find it helpful to 'fill in the gaps' or copy the statements that are provided in the template, other people find it restricting. If this is the case for you, adapt the wording to make it *meaningful* to your situation – hopefully you can see the general direction of the statements provided and can then work out how you would say or write it in your own words.

If you have found adopting a particular posture helpful it may be useful to use this posture in all future exercises, not just while letter writing.

As part of your regular 'self-practice' it may be helpful to use this exercise often, but instead of looking at your situation in 'general' terms, think about it over the last 24 hours or week. An example of such a letter can be found below.

Jenny's story

Jenny worked at the local supermarket. She had passed by job promotions time and time again, saying to her employers that she was happy, for the time being, with her present role. Underneath, promotion filled her with dread. She feared she wouldn't be able to do the things required of her and would make a hash of it. Gradually, as Jenny developed her self-confidence, she took on a few more new opportunities at work. Then, when her supervisor was taken ill she was asked to take her role temporarily. Jenny surprised herself by agreeing and felt proud that she had both been asked and had accepted the position. Although at certain times she felt overwhelmed, her new role was really rewarding. However, when a further colleague went on long-term sick Jenny's workload suddenly increased. Over the course of a week she found she had made a few silly errors, ones she would never have previously made. Jenny felt waves of anxiety. To address the return of her self-criticism she was able to use compassionate imagery and soothing rhythm breathing over the remainder of the week.

That weekend, Jenny recalled the mistakes she had made and once again she felt a wave of anxiety. On noting this she went to her room and, sitting quietly, engaged in her soothing rhythm breathing. She then opened her journal and wrote:

It is understandable that I have found it difficult to build my self-confidence this week because there have been a whole number of new things happening at work, I have been pushed into new roles and such things have activated my fears of failing...........This was really tough...........

In the past I have coped by trying to get out of things, taking time off or even taking beta blockers, but all of these things prevented me from building my self-confidence. But recently I decided to give things a go properly, despite my concerns. This took a lot of guts and I am glad I did it, despite finding it difficult. I used imagery exercises to help me accept the fact that I was anxious and this also helped me believe that the mistakes I made did not mean that I was useless. I even told a couple of people I was anxious, and amazingly this really helped as I felt supported by them.

Now, standing back from things, I can see that in actual fact my self-confidence has grown this week. Maybe the best weeks for learning are the ones I also find difficult. In the future it would help if I did what I did today. It would also help if I reminded myself that there was a positive outcome this week.

Exercise 41: Compassionate letter writing from the compassionate role to yourself

Prepare for this exercise in the way you have previously found most helpful.

Now put pen to paper and write a supportive letter to yourself from the perspective of a compassionate role.[20] Your letter could be focused on something very *specific*, such as how you are feeling right now, or a situation that recently happened. Alternatively it could take a more *general* stance with respect to how you view yourself. It may open with a

---

[20] Because people prefer to use different imagery to evoke a compassionate mindset, here we will refer to the 'compassionate role', be it the ideal compassionate self, the perfect nurturer or the compassionate coach/teacher.

statement such as 'I am sorry that you are having a difficult time at the moment and are struggling to build your self-confidence............'

Tracey's story

Tracey's family were often critical of her. At a family gathering she had watched as her nephew, Ben, was poked fun at by his uncle. Her nephew clearly looked upset. After taking a calming breath, Tracey remarked 'Don't be cruel, Paul', but instead of having the desired effect her comment was met by a barrage of criticism directed towards her. Tracey turned round and walked away, taking her nephew with her. That evening Tracey wrote:

I am sorry that today has been really difficult for you. Being around certain people can be tough. It is understandable that you feel a whole range of emotions such as frustration, anger, anxiety and sadness, given what happened. This is a difficult environment in which to build your self-confidence. But it would be helpful for you to acknowledge that you did volunteer your opinion and this took courage. People are complicated and sometimes it is helpful just to acknowledge that. Maybe they don't see what an impact this is having on you. Together we will build your self-confidence; I have your back through good times and set-backs. Each day you find out more about yourself and this will help you grow.

When you feel that you have completed your letter, put down your pen or pencil and for a few moments engage in one of the exercises aimed at evoking a compassionate frame of mind.

Now, when you feel ready, slowly re-read your letter. Engage with the emotion that the letter conveys rather than focusing on how you have written it, the grammar, words or phrasing.

Once you have done this, allow yourself to sit for a while, feeling a sense of warmth and allowing the exercise to 'sink in'.

Reflection on Exercise 41

You may have noticed that when you are writing letters, either a 'you' or an 'I' approach works better for you. Some people, however, find it makes no difference. It may be helpful to you to experiment further with these two options and see which helps you best in different situations.

Exercise 42: Writing a compassionate letter based on a compassionate alternative thoughts/images worksheet

In this exercise you will use one of your compassionate alternative thoughts/images worksheets from the last chapter as a focus. Having already gained experience from the exercises so far, you may now decide to focus on a thought or image that is associated with strong emotions. Alternatively you may decide to start with one that is less challenging. The choice is yours.

First, re-familiarize yourself with the worksheet and have it close at hand.

Prepare for the exercise in any manner you have found helpful previously.

Now review your chosen worksheet. To begin with, focus on the column containing your undermining thoughts and images and begin to write compassionately about such things.

Alan's story

Upon entering work, Alan was met by his boss who asked him to present some information at a meeting later that afternoon. This was something he had never done before and understandably he felt overwhelmed. Having completed a compassionate alternative thoughts/images worksheet during the day, that evening he wrote:

I am sorry that you often feel that you can't cope in situations. When you were put on the spot at work it is understandable that you panicked. This then led you to feel upset and self-critical. You often tell yourself you are pathetic in these situations and this goes back to school days when you were bullied............

It is hoped that this part of the letter will be sensitive to the difficulties you have and validate the associated emotions.

When you feel that you have focused on the first column for long enough, allow yourself time to review what you have written so far and let it 'sink in'. Now turn your attention to the alternative thoughts and images column.

Alan went on to write: *It may be helpful to remind myself that I never totally screw up. In addition I have a tendency to focus on the negative (like everyone else does to some extent), and as I recall there were things that went well, such as............*

Because of the experiences I have had, I have learnt to be critical of myself but I am now learning that it is more helpful to be self-compassionate and nurture myself by............My compassionate coach knows that I am doing my best...... ......I am doing my best............I am a human being who struggles............ many other people also struggle – it's not just me.

Take time to explore in your own letter all the work you did previously on the worksheet. When you feel as though your letter is complete, put your pen down for a few moments and engage once more in one of the centring exercises you find helpful. This may be a mindfulness exercise, soothing rhythm breathing or some form of imagery.

After a short while re-read your letter slowly. You may prefer to read it out loud or in your head.

Once you have done this, sit for a while, feeling a sense of warmth and allowing the exercise to 'sink in'.

Reflection on Exercise 42

It is hoped that this specific letter-writing exercise will help to consolidate the work you have already done on the compassionate alternative thoughts/images worksheets. You may now decide to focus on other worksheets you have completed, and perhaps regularly write a letter every time you complete a new one. I personally find it most beneficial to use the compassionate alternative thought worksheets in response to things that have triggered strong emotions or feelings of self-criticism in me. In other words, I tend to use them in a *reactive* way. Then, once a week, I *proactively* write a compassionate letter to myself, perhaps using a recent worksheet as the basis for it.

Reviewing Your Compassionate Letters

Once you have completed a letter it is a good idea to review it using the guiding principles found on page 179. This can help to enhance your letter and its focus. Do this in a frame of mind which holds curiosity and warmth, rather than one that is judgemental and cold.

As a starting point, each of the guiding principles found on page 179 can be turned into questions. For example, was your letter sensitive to, and did it validate, the emotions you experienced? Did it convey understanding, acceptance and caring? Did it validate the reasons why you may be struggling with certain things?

Secondly, does your letter capture a sense of warmth throughout? If you noticed that parts of it contain less warmth, or are cold or even hostile, it may be worth warmly reflecting on why this may be. For example:

Did your self-critic step in?

Did you feel as though you were 'kidding yourself'?

Were you undermining your own efforts?

Was your drive or threat system 'kicking in', making statements such as 'you should do X' and 'you shouldn't do Y'?

All such observations are very helpful as they direct us towards further avenues of exploration. Depending on the particular obstacle you notice, it may help you to engage in an imagery exercise focusing on this difficulty or else to complete a compassionate alternative thoughts/images worksheet focusing on these specific thoughts and images.

As a further exercise, many people find it helpful to write a letter looking specifically at the obstacle itself.

For example, Peter found letter writing difficult. He wrote: *At times when I write in this way I start telling myself I need to 'get a grip'. I get frustrated with myself and think the struggling part of me is pathetic. Reflecting upon where this comes from, I know that this is related to how I was treated in the past and that I have learnt to do it to myself. It may be helpful for me to recall the story of which teacher I would send my child to. Of course I would choose the compassionate teacher for David (son), and this is the teacher it would be helpful for me to approach myself, instead of the critical one. Through being compassionate to myself I will gain strength and courage and reduce my tendency to judge myself.*

Adaptations to Compassionate Letter Writing

Here are some of the many ways people have used and enhanced their own compassionate letter writing. It may be worth trying some of these modifications for yourself:

• Write different parts of your letter in different-coloured pens to emphasize different points.

• Record your letters, remembering to use a warm compassionate tone, and then play them back at different times when you are in need of compassion, maybe at the beginning or end of the day.

• Read a letter aloud to yourself in front of a mirror, again remembering to use a warm compassionate tone.

• Read a letter while focusing on a photograph of yourself. Depending upon what the letter is about, it may help you to use a photograph of yourself as a child or as an adult. Sometimes holding a photo of yourself taken at a particular time, maybe when things were most difficult for you, can have a very powerful effect.

• Add pictures, photographs and drawings to your letters in order to increase their emotional impact.

- Write out complete or parts of longer letters on the back of post-cards chosen to convey a sense of warmth, and carry them with you.

- Scent your letters with something that evokes a sense of warmth and soothing. This may be a perfume, aftershave or aromatherapy oil. Enjoy 'sniffing around' to find something that is helpful for you.

- Use a specific chair, as you did in Chapter 10, to help evoke your compassionate mind, and write while sitting in this chair.

- Sit in a chair and allow yourself to become in touch with difficult feelings surrounding a situation (past, present or future). Once you have experienced and written about these feelings, move to a second chair, allowing yourself to step outside the previous feelings and to reflect on them, then write from your new perspective.

- Sit in a chair and evoke your ideal compassionate self or compassionate image, such as your compassionate coach or companion. Remind yourself of all of their qualities and attributes. Now, facing a second chair, read out one of your letters. Then move to the second chair and experience what was said.

- Read your letters at different times of the day and before or after certain events to see if this is helpful to you.

- Look out for positive things (such as events, things people have said, how they have behaved or things you have realized) during the day and make a note of them in order that you can use this as material for your next letter.

- Write a letter to your inner self-critic, acknowledging that they may have your welfare at heart but telling them they are going about things the wrong way. Explain to them what you need from them in order to build your self-confidence.

- Write a letter to people in the past who might have hurt you, on purpose or not, telling them how you felt then and how you feel now. This can be an emotional exercise so remember to evoke inner strength, support, wisdom and courage, from an imagery or breathing exercise.

- Write a letter to yourself as a younger person. What messages and emotions does your compassionate mind want the child or the younger adult to hear and feel?

- Write a letter to yourself from an older, wiser compassionate you. What would you say to yourself now and what would a compassionate future look like?

Conclusions

Compassionate letter writing can be an extremely powerful, emotional and beneficial exercise. As you can see, there are a number of ways that you can adapt it or combine it with other ideas. Be creative and develop something that works for you.

It may be beneficial to engage in letter writing, as well as re-reading letters, every week or even every day initially. Later it may be helpful to develop this into something that becomes an integral part of your life.

In the next chapter we will draw upon some of the ideas generated in your compassionate letters. They will provide the focus for some new exercises aimed at 'taking action' to increase compassionate behaviour.

12 Taking Action – Compassionate Behaviour

It is worth reflecting that all the work you have done so far, from initially picking up this book to reading it, engaging in exercises and developing your own practice, *is* in fact self-compassionate behaviour. However, the next two chapters will focus on how you may take further action to build your self-confidence by:

- Generating your own personal goals

- Identifying the steps you need to take

- Preparing for taking action by:

    (i)   using compassionate imagery

    (ii) using compassionate letter writing

    (iii) using a compassionate alternative thoughts/images worksheet

    (iv) using compassionate behavioural experiment worksheets

- Taking action

- Reviewing compassionate behavioural experiments and learning from them

Each of the exercises covered in this chapter is listed on your personal practice summary sheet on page xxx. It may be helpful to you to use this as a place in which to record your reflections on and summaries of the exercises – as well, of course, as continuing to use your journal or notebook.

'We gain strength, and courage, and confidence by each experience in which we really stop to look fear in the face ... we must do that which we think we cannot'

– Eleanor Roosevelt

Generating Your Own Personal Goals and Breaking Them Down into Manageable Steps

Building on all your previous work, it is important to focus on generating your goals from a compassionate mindset. In other words, you should *warmly* choose to work towards things that will be of benefit to you. (This is in contrast to responding to self-criticism, or that of others, by deciding on things because you 'should' or 'have to'.)

Here is a range of goals that other people wanting to build their self-confidence have worked towards previously. As you can see, there are many different things that you could focus on, such as:

Meeting new people

Public speaking

Being comfortable handing in pieces of work that are not perfect

Being able to put your point of view across to others – be they people you know well or those you don't

Putting yourself forward for job opportunities

Doing things just for pleasure

Being able to ask for help

Being able to apologize

Stopping apologizing needlessly

Being able to assert yourself in difficult relationships

Being able to tell people how you feel

Being able to take back faulty goods or things you decide against

Saying no to people

Saying yes to people

Exercise 43: Identifying your own personal goals with respect to building your self-confidence

Find a place where you can be, as far as possible, free from major distractions for 5–10 minutes. Sit in a relaxed, open posture that has *strength* or *alertness* in it. Close your eyes or settle your gaze on a low fixed point.

Engage in your soothing rhythm breathing or use your place of contentment imagery and experience a sense of soothing. Now bring to mind your chosen compassionate image, maybe your compassionate coach, teacher, companion or nurturer. Alternatively evoke the sense of your ideal compassionate self. Remind yourself of the key compassionate qualities. Feel a sense of strength, courage and warmth, and allow a slight smile to appear on your face.

Now, in this frame of mind, ask yourself what goals it would be helpful for you to work towards – goals that will help you build your self-confidence.

If it is difficult for you to generate these goals, it may be worth reflecting on times in the past when you have lacked self-confidence. What was the situation, what happened, and what would you have done differently then if you had been more self-confident? What would you change about yourself in the situation?

When you are ready, use the space provided overleaf to write down some specific goals that you wish to work towards.

When you are happy with your list, place numbers next to each of the goals you have identified. Start by putting the number 1 against the goal that you think will be the most difficult, then the number 2 against the goal you think is slightly less difficult, and so forth until you have numbered all of the goals. The text box overleaf has some tips to help you.

James's story (page 200) summarises how he used exercises 43 and 44 to identify and break down his goals into manageable steps.

My goals are:	Difficulty rating

....

....

....

....

....

....

....

....

....

....

....

....

....

....

Additional hint:

It is highly likely that the formulation you drew out in Chapter 4 will give you some ideas for things you wish to work towards. For example, in the 'coping strategies' box you may have identified a number of things that have unintended consequences or drawbacks. When Andy reviewed his formulation (pages 61 and 184) he was able to generate a number of additional goals, such as being himself with others/opening up, engaging in social activities he usually ignored and reducing how much alcohol he drank.

You may find it helpful to ask someone you trust, someone who has your best interests at heart, for their thoughts. They may be able to generate some goals with you.

Further ideas could be drawn from the exercises you have done previously and your personal notes and reflections. It may be helpful to review these.

Exercise 44: Identifying the steps you need to take in working towards a goal

Starting with the goal you have identified as the 'least difficult', you are now going to identify some simple steps that will help you achieve it. You can set yourself as many steps as you see fit. By doing so, you will break down the task into manageable stages, which will make it seem less overwhelming. Once again, it will be helpful to you to adopt a compassionate mindset when approaching this exercise.

Below you will see how James followed this process to help him achieve one of his goals.

If, however, you feel as though you are ready to tackle the least difficult goal straight away, without breaking it down into smaller steps in this way, go ahead and do so – but remember the technique of setting yourself stages when dealing with further goals that are more difficult to achieve.

My goal is:

Step 1:..

Step 2:..

Step 3:..

Step 4:..

Step 5:..

Step 6:..

James's story

James was 24 and two years previously had got his dream job working at a very junior level in a busy law firm. His self-confidence was low but he knew that if he wished to progress in his chosen career he would have to address this. Although James felt self-confident with his friends and family, his confidence often failed him at work and with strangers. His list of initial goals can be found below:

Goal	Difficulty rating
Being able to contribute ideas/thoughts at work	3
Getting on a busy underground train	2
Putting myself forward for the next round of promotions	1
Taking on a mentee at work	4
Being able to ask a stranger for directions	6
Taking something back to a shop	5

As you can see from the goals listed above, James identified that the 'easiest' goal for him to achieve was being able to ask strangers for directions. This goal was important to him as he often had to make deliveries on foot to law firms. The thought of asking someone for directions filled him with dread. All sorts of thoughts ran through his head and undermined his self-confidence, such as 'They will think I am an idiot', 'They will see I am anxious' and 'If I can't get this simple thing right, I am pathetic'.

With the help of one of his close friends James generated a number of steps. Each was designed to help him advance further towards achieving his goal.

How James broke down his goal into easy steps

My goal is: Being able to ask a stranger for directions

Step 1: Walk to the local high street at a quiet time and ask someone who seems approachable

a) where the nearest chemist is

b) where Burton Road is

c) where the station is

Repeat 3 times

Step 2: Go into a busy street and ask someone

a) where the nearest chemist is

b) where Oxford Road is

c) where the train station is

Repeat 3 times

Step 3: Go at peak time and repeat step 2

Step 4: Repeat steps 2 and 3 but this time approach someone who looks busy or not approachable

Step 5: While making a delivery at work, to somewhere you know, check out with a stranger that you are going to the right place

Repeat 3 times

Step 6: Next time you are making a delivery at work and need directions, ask a stranger for them

Reflection on Exercises 43 and 44

You can plan as many goals and associated steps as you want and, of course, the things you are planning are not set in stone. Many people modify the number of stages as they become more familiar with the process.

You may have been able to do these exercises very quickly or you may need to think them through and add to them over a few days. What is important is that you proceed to the next exercise only when you feel ready.

Some people find that rather than being 'happy' with their list of goals to accomplish they are daunted by it, while others find that they avoid putting down certain steps or goals because they think they are far too difficult or are associated with strong emotions. Remember, we are aiming to build your self-confidence step by step. You will proceed at your own pace and set yourself easy-to-achieve goals to begin with.

'Courage is not the absence of fear, but rather the judgment that something is more important than fear'

– Ambrose Hollingworth Redmoon

Preparing to Take Action

In this section I will outline a range of different ways you can further prepare yourself to take action to build your self-confidence, in both social and non-social situations, using a variety of techniques from imagery to compassionate letter writing.

Exercise 45: Preparing to take action in social situations: using compassionate imagery I

This exercise is designed to prepare you specifically for building self-confidence in situations that involve other people.

When we are lacking in self-confidence we can fall into a number of traps that stop us from thinking about a situation as a whole. For example, many people report that in social situations they feel as though they are being singled out in some way – as if everyone is looking at them. Others view themselves totally through the eyes of other people. When we are lacking in self-confidence we often believe we are acting in an unacceptable or disappointing way and that other people are scrutinizing and appraising us negatively.

You may already be aware of imagery strategies designed to help with such situations. For example, by imagining interviewers, audience members or assessors in their underwear, or else sitting on the toilet, as a means of reducing anxiety. This strategy is aimed at 'bringing everyone to the same level' and can help in situations where you feel intimidated, scrutinized and judged.

Although this strategy may already be helpful to you, in this exercise you will be asked to use a compassionate image (maybe your perfect nurturer, compassionate coach or companion) or ideal compassionate self to help change your perspective on a social situation.

James's story continued

James, for example, *knew* that people wouldn't think he was stupid when he asked for directions, but he still *felt* as though they thought badly of him when he needed to ask for assistance.

In preparation for taking his first step towards increasing his self-confidence, James brought to mind his ideal compassionate self and reminded himself of their qualities and attributes. He felt a sense of warmth and a gentle smile on his face. Inhabiting this image, he imagined himself engaging in the first step from his list (page 201). He imagined himself standing on his local high street as people passed by. He imagined a middle-aged man thinking about his day ahead and rushing by, an older man reciting his shopping list to himself, a postwoman delivering letters, a family on their way to the bus, a teenager listening to music as she passed by. In turn he imagined what was going on for them, what was running through their minds.

Then he imagined himself asking these people for directions to the nearest chemist. From his compassionate frame of mind he reflected on what each person might think as they were interrupted in this way. He imagined that one person felt abruptly forced out of their daydreaming and 'put on the spot' since they could not think where the chemist's was; another felt slightly annoyed that they had to stop for a moment, another did not seem to think anything, another felt positive about having a brief interaction with someone.

This exercise helped James prepare for the experiment he was planning in a few days' time.

Now it's your turn. Prepare for this exercise in the manner you have found most helpful previously. When you are ready, bring to mind your chosen compassionate image or else evoke the sense of your ideal compassionate self. Remind yourself of the key compassionate qualities. Feel a sense of strength and warmth, and allow a slight smile to appear on your face.

Now imagine the social situation you are preparing for. Imagine yourself in the situation. If you are imagining yourself as your ideal compassionate self, see the situation from this new perspective. If you bring to mind a compassionate image, imagine that the coach, companion or nurturer is supporting you in this situation. Draw a sense of strength and courage from them.

Now turn your attention to the other people in the scene. Individual by individual, ask yourself what the other people there are likely to be experiencing. What are they thinking? Attempt to take a comprehensive and compassionate view of their feelings.

If you notice that your threat system is activated, and you start to feel strong emotions such as anxiety or anger, return to the soothing rhythm breathing or imagery exercise you did in preparation. Remind yourself of the key compassionate qualities of strength, courage and wisdom. When you are ready, resume the exercise.

When you feel you have explored this situation as best you can, gently let the image fade and return to your compassionate image or ideal compassionate self. Engage in your soothing rhythm breathing again if this is helpful.

After a few minutes, gently bring your awareness to the end of the exercise and become more aware of your physical environment.

Exercise 46: Preparing to take action: using compassionate imagery II

This exercise is similar to the preceding one but can be used for both social and non-social situations.

Engage in your soothing rhythm breathing or using your place of contentment imagery to promote a sense of soothing. When you are ready, bring to mind your chosen compassionate image or evoke the sense of your ideal compassionate self. Remind yourself of the key qualities of compassion. Feel a sense of warmth and allow a slight smile to appear on your face.

Now imagine the situation you are preparing for. Picture yourself in the situation. If you are imagining yourself as your ideal compassionate self, see the situation from this new perspective. If you bring to mind a compassionate image, imagine that the coach, companion or nurturer is supporting you in this situation. Feel a sense of strength and courage from them.

Now, observe yourself having successfully completed the task. Imagine how this feels, in your mind and in your body. This feeling may be one of strength or excitement, you may feel a broadening across your chest or a sense of warmth. Now observe yourself doing the task, feeling a sense of strength and courage. If you can imagine yourself suffering a setback, take time to experience the support provided by your ideal compassionate self or compassionate image.

Spend some time imagining the scene. Where appropriate, use your senses to make the scene 'come to life'. What do you smell? What can you see? What sounds can you hear? What kind of helpful thoughts and images might occupy your mind in this situation?

Once you feel as though you have explored this imagery sufficiently, return to your soothing rhythm breathing or your compassionate imagery and let the scene fade from your mind.

After a few minutes gently bring your awareness to the end of the exercise and become more aware of your physical environment.

Hazel's story

Hazel had self-confidence in a range of situations but she found doing things on her own very difficult. She wasn't in a relationship and desperately wanted to go on holiday – something she thought she would never be able to do on her own. When the company she worked for was taken over, she had the opportunity to add a holiday on to a trip to Canada she needed to make for work. None of her friends was free to go along so this meant that she had to decide whether to go on her own or not at all.

Some of Hazel's concerns centred around what people would make of her being on her own. She thought they would pity her, think she must be weird and have no friends. Other worries were concerned with being in 'the great outdoors' on her own, and being on her own in her hostel room at night. Compassionate alternative thought worksheets had been useful to her previously when dealing with her own lack of self-confidence, and Hazel decided to use them again to prepare herself for this challenge.

She booked the holiday and, in the weeks leading up to it, set herself some smaller steps to help her feel more self-confident. Among other things, she decided to go for a picnic on her own into the local countryside, go to the cinema to see an obscure film (at a time when she knew there wouldn't be people she knew around) and plan a night away at a hostel not too far from where she lived.

Before each of these activities Hazel imagined herself into the situation in the company of her compassionate coach. She imagined them supporting and encouraging her, which helped her evoke a sense of strength and courage prior to taking each new step. When the step involved interacting with other people she also used her compassionate mindset to imagine what might be in their minds at the time, a technique she found very helpful. After doing this for only a short time Hazel was already starting to feel empowered. She noticed that in situations she had previously found daunting, even without conscious effort she was better able to draw on her inner strength, her posture changed and she actually found herself enjoying the new experiences she had set herself to accomplish. The more she practised, and the more steps she took, the more her self-confidence grew. The final tasks she had set herself were actually easier to achieve than the first few, and, though still occasionally anxious, the anticipation she experienced prior to new situations was almost a pleasurable feeling rather than a crippling one.

Reflection on Exercises 45 and 46

Because these exercises require you to imagine yourself in difficult situations you may experience some uncomfortable feelings while you perform them. This is perfectly normal. When you notice difficult feelings, thoughts and physical sensations, be mindful of them. If it helps, return to your soothing rhythm breathing or compassionate imagery. Once you are more centred, resume the exercise.

Some people report initial feelings of scepticism about the usefulness of these exercises. However, time and time again people report that once they are *in* the situation, having prepared for it in this way helps them maintain a broader perspective. They feel supported and become less focused on feelings of threat or insecurity.

Exercise 47: Preparing to take action: using a compassionate alternative thoughts/images worksheet

The compassionate mind approach aims to build your self-confidence by developing a range of strategies and techniques that can be used successively, collectively, or, at times, in isolation. If you find that obstacles to your progress arise in the form of negative thoughts or images it may be helpful to you to return to Chapter 10 and use the compassionate alternative thoughts/images worksheets there to help you resolve this.

Exercise 48: Preparing to take action: accessing inner support using compassionate letter writing

By now you may have a preferred way of preparing to write a compassionate letter. This may involve sitting in a certain place at a specific time with a particular pen and diary/journal. You may first use a mindfulness, breathing or imagery exercise to evoke a compassionate frame of mind and this may be supplemented by using a particular scent, piece of music or other such strategy. Whatever way you prepare to engage in this exercise, what is important is to use the prompts that are most helpful to you.

Now, from the perspective of the ideal compassionate self, your compassionate coach, companion or perfect nurturer, put pen to paper and write a supportive letter to yourself in preparation for the action you are planning to take. It would help if the letter acknowledges the difficult thing you are aiming to do, wishes you the strength and courage to see it through, and reminds you that this is a new chapter in your life where you can experiment with situations and find out more about your inner strength and capabilities.

For example, before Hazel went for a picnic on her own she wrote:

What you are planning to do tomorrow is going to be difficult, but you will get through it. Of course you are going to be anxious............breathe and observe the anxiety as it increases and decreases............try not to get caught up in it. If you get overly anxious, try to remember that it's not your fault............ it may help to do an imagery exercise or soothing rhythm breathing. This is one step further towards your holiday to Canada which is likely to be one of the most empowering things you have done to date in your life. This is a step further towards a new, more self-confident you.

As you have seen, compassionate letters can take all sorts of forms. Here Hazel wrote as if someone were cheering her on, and being encouraging yet supportive however the experiment turned out. It may be helpful to look at the guiding principles for compassionate letter writing in Chapter 11 (page 176) again to help you with this exercise.

Exercise 49: Preparing to take action: compassionate behavioural experiment worksheets

So far we have identified your goals, broken them down into steps and then used imagery plus maybe compassionate alternative thought worksheets and compassionate letter writing to help you prepare for taking action. We will now focus on using a compassionate behavioural experiment worksheet in final preparation.

These worksheets help clarify what you are about to do and remind you of why it may be helpful to take such action. They help you anticipate obstacles and ways of dealing with them. While some people find that they easily complete a worksheet such as this in a self-supporting style, others find that spending a little time engaging in breathing or imagery exercises prior to tackling it helps them undertake it in a compassionate mindset.

Now it is time to use worksheet 8 on page 210 in final preparation for 'taking action' to build your self-confidence. Take time to reflect on each section. There is a worked example on page 212 relating to James's experiences to act as a guide.

Worksheet 8: Compassionate behavioural experiment worksheet

The step I am now going to take is: _____

_____

The things I can do to help me prepare for this are: _____

_____

_____

_____

_____

_____

_____

_____

The potential obstacles I can see are:

_____

_____

_____

_____

_____

_____

_____

I can do the following things to help me negotiate the obstacles:

_____

_____

_____

_____

_____

_____

_____

The things it would be helpful for me to remember just before and during the situation are:

_____

_____

_____

_____

_____

_____

_____

_____

_____

The additional things I can do to help me in the situation are:

_____

_____

_____

_____

_____

_____

_____

_____

_____

The things it would be helpful to tell myself after I have taken this step are:

_____

_____

_____

_____

_____

_____

_____

_____

_____

James's example

In order to prepare himself for a compassionate behavioural experiment James completed the following worksheet.

The step I am now going to take is:

to go to the high street and ask for directions.

The things I can do to help me prepare for this are:

Use compassionate imagery – both in relation to seeing people from a different perspective and in evoking a sense of strength from my compassionate coach.

When I write a compassionate letter to myself tonight, I will use it as an opportunity to reflect on what I am about to do.

I will also arrange to see one of my friends this evening so, no matter how it goes, I will have something to look forward to.

Before I go out I will have a shower and make sure I have something I feel comfortable and confident in to wear – both things generally make me feel better about myself.

The potential obstacles I can see are:

I may start to panic and become lost for words.

People may ignore me.

I may chicken out.

I can do the following things to help me negotiate the obstacles:

I can use my soothing rhythm breathing if I get panicky.

I can do some mindfulness and/or imagery exercises.

If people ignore me, I can tell myself it may be nothing to do with me.

I can tell myself that not everyone is going to be friendly and concentrate my efforts on finding someone who is helpful.

If I find the urge to avoid the situation I can remind myself that this is just an experiment and a step further towards the things I want to achieve in life.

The things it would be helpful for me to remember just before and during the situation are:

This is going to help me learn about myself – whichever way it goes, it will help me develop my self-confidence because I will know more at the end of it.

Afterwards I can give myself a pat on the back for facing the things I am fearful of.

I can always revert to my soothing rhythm breathing/take a break/ use some imagery if it is difficult.

Other people struggle as I do – it's not just me.

There are many things that I can do – it is good to bring them to mind.

The additional things I can do to help me in the situation are:

I can assume a relaxed and open yet confident posture.

Having previously used the manipulation of a smooth pebble to help me in some of the imagery exercises, I will put it in my pocket to help me if difficult situations arise.

The things it would be helpful to tell myself after I have taken this step are:

Whatever the outcome, facing this is an achievement – it shows I have courage.

It is OK to renegotiate the steps and rethink things if they don't go to plan.

If things don't go to plan, I will at least know more and can then go through this process again.

This is worth the effort I am putting in – no matter what the outcome is.

Building something is hard and takes time.

I can be proud of myself if I attempt to do this.

Reflection on Exercises 48 and 49

Some people find that these preparatory exercises are best done in the order set out in this chapter while others prefer doing things in a different sequence. Choose whatever works best for you.

Although I would recommend that you have a go at them all, if you find you can't resist the urge to design an experiment and do it instead, that is OK too. It may be that you find that you need little preparation in the early stages but more as you work up to more difficult tests of your self-confidence. Alternatively, some people find that the early exercises help prepare them for the later ones, so there is less of a build-up required later on.

Doing and Reviewing

Finally you have reached the part of the book that involves 'doing' or experimenting with situations. It is hoped that you will already have experienced changes in your level of self-confidence but this stage marks a significant advance.

Exercise 50: Doing your compassionate behavioural experiment

Compassionate behavioural experiments are exactly that – experiments. If possible, view them as a means to find out more about yourself and/or other people. Remember, *information is power*. Ironically, the steps you take here are likely to be incredibly big ones and yet this is the shortest section of the chapter, if not the book!

Exercise 51: Reviewing your compassionate behavioural experiment

The following worksheet can be used to review the action you have taken in your compassionate behavioural experiment. It may be helpful first to complete the worksheet below in a spontaneous way, then revisit it having practised an exercise that evokes a compassionate frame of mind, such as imagery or soothing rhythm breathing. This new perspective may enable you to write additional entries on your sheet. An example completed by Hazel can also be found on page 217, to illustrate how it can best be used.

Worksheet 9 : My reflections on my compassionate behavioural experiment

The step I took was: _____

_____

How did the exercise go in general?_____

_____

_____

_____

_____

The things I learnt about myself through the exercise were: _____

_____

_____

The things I learnt about other people through the exercise were [optional depending on the action taken]:

_____

_____

_____

_____

_____

_____

_____

The things it would be helpful for me to remember just before and during such situations are: _____

_____

_____

_____

_____

_____

_____

_____

The potential adjustments that I could make to myself or the situation in the future are: _____

_____

_____

_____

_____

_____

_____

_____

In summary: _____

_____

_____

_____

_____

_____

_____

Taking all of this into account, it may be helpful for me to do the following in order to build my self-confidence further: _____

_____

_____

_____

_____

Hazel's example

The step I took was: to stay a night in a hostel on my own

How did the exercise go in general?:

Things went well. I was really anxious at first, but I got to my room and settled in. I met some people in the communal area who seemed nice. Some were with other people, some were on their own. There just seemed to be an 'acceptance' from everyone regarding what other people were doing/why they were there.

There was one girl who seemed a bit aloof but I then engaged with some imagery exercises and that helped me think about what might be going on for her – she might have been anxious herself or maybe not interested in talking, and that is OK.

Breakfast was a bit awkward as I ended up sitting by myself as there was no room on the larger table but I read my book and practised some mindfulness exercises.

The things I learnt about myself through the exercise were:

Although it was anxiety-provoking at times, I proved that I can do it.

I have more courage than I thought.

I can enjoy time on my own – it was quite liberating.

The things I learnt about other people through the exercise were:

Other people stay at hostels on their own.

People did not seem to judge me in any way.

A group of girls ended up chatting to me in the kitchen and said they had met up while travelling alone.

People are nicer than I thought – in actual fact there were other people like me.

There are always going to be people around that I don't get on with – that is normal.

The things it would be helpful for me to remember just before and during the situation are:

All of the above, but in addition – it is worthwhile experimenting with situations.

Experimenting is actually quite exciting.

Things hardly ever go perfectly but they can still be worthwhile nevertheless.

At this moment in time I feel a lot more confident – this will fade but I need to savour it and remind myself of this just before I put myself in another situation.

The potential adjustments that I could make to myself or the situation in the future are:

When I stay in a hostel again it may be good to go into the communal areas more often – maybe sitting and reading, maybe chatting.

I don't need to explain myself – if people ask, I could maybe just say, 'Yes, I am travelling alone, none of my friends could get the leave.'

It's OK to stay in my room as well, if I feel like it. It doesn't make me sad, it just makes me human.

In summary:

This exercise was so liberating – I am so glad I did it. The experiment allowed me to visit a different place and have a great experience – yes, it was difficult at times but that is OK – it is the first time I have done it and I can learn from it – making the next visit better. I can cope with anxiety-provoking situations and they don't have to stop me living my life.

Taking all of this into account it may be helpful for me to do the following in order to build my self-confidence further:

Stay at another hostel for a weekend, somewhere less familiar.

Tell people that I have been away for a weekend by myself, staying in a hostel, and see what they say – evoke strength and courage from my compassionate coach before I tell them so I can feel empowered, as opposed to awkward and apologetic – after all, it was fun and even if I had offers of company I may still decide to do it on my own at times.

Courage does not always roar. Sometimes courage is the quiet voice at the end of the day, saying, 'I will try again tomorrow'

– *Mary Anne Radmacher*

Reflection on Exercise 51

It may be helpful to use the worksheet exactly as it is, or you may wish to customize it. Either is fine. In addition you may find it helpful to use this material as the basis for a compassionate letter. Have a go and see if this helps.

Conclusions

In this chapter we have looked at 'taking action' by means of compassionate behaviour. In fact all the things you have done so far in this book could also be classed as this, but the exercises outlined in this chapter will hopefully have helped you make additional self-compassionate behavioural changes that will help build your self-confidence.

In the next chapter we will look at some other ways to help you 'take action', such as assertiveness techniques and making small (or big) changes to your everyday life that may be of further benefit to you.

13 Additional Strategies to Help Build Your Self-confidence

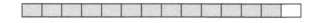

In this penultimate chapter we will review a number of additional ways to help you build your self-confidence. The chapter will cover:

- Assertiveness strategies

- Small behavioural changes

- Savouring positive experiences

- Acceptance

- Using self-compassion to guide your day

- Using self-compassion to help you *in* difficult situations

Consistent with the general approach of this book, it is possible for some of the following exercises to be used in combination with others you have already tried, as a means of enhancing them. Alternatively the exercises may be used in isolation. The important thing is to give things a go and find something that is effective for you.

Each of the exercises covered in this chapter can be found on your personal practice summary sheet on page xxxi. It may be helpful to use this as a space for reflection and summary, which will be of help to you when working through the final chapter of the book.

Assertiveness Strategies

Being assertive means being able to express ourselves while also being respectful of the views, feelings and needs of others. This may include expressing our emotions, needs and points of view. When we assertively express ourselves we are being neither apologetic nor aggressive. Assertiveness is about finding a state in between. While some people who struggle with assertiveness fluctuate between two extremes (for example, aggressive then submissive), others find that they almost always follow the same pattern – tending to one or the other every time.

Sometimes people think that in order to be assertive they must *know* how they are feeling, have a clear point of view or be able to identify a specific need. However, at times assertiveness means expressing a mixture of emotions. It can involve stating 'I don't know', 'don't care' or 'don't know what I need'. Equally, assertiveness may be deciding not to show our emotions, share our views, thoughts and needs if we don't want to do so – confusing, isn't it? Basically assertiveness is about us acknowledging how we think, how we feel, what we need and what we want to do – and in the process respecting ourselves and others.

Assertiveness can be a consequence of, or can help build, self-confidence. It is a learned skill and one that we can develop. I hope that some of the exercises covered so far will have helped you build your own capacity to be assertive. For example, it is hoped that to date you have gained a better understanding of yourself, as well as of others. Understanding our situation, and that of other people, can help us feel less ashamed and more empowered.

It is hoped that the mindfulness exercises, soothing rhythm breathing, and in particular the imagery exercises have already given you a sense of strength and courage. In addition, work on the thoughts and images that play out in your head, letter writing, and especially the compassionate behavioural experiments, are also likely to have improved your ability to assert yourself.

In this section we will look at a couple of exercises that will hopefully enhance this. The first will focus on how to give others feedback relating to how you feel. The second will involve how to give those around us feedback in general.

Before we look at the exercises, Sarah's story will illustrate how difficulties asserting oneself can lead to all manner of problems.

Sarah's story

Sarah used to feel that she was not taken seriously at work. Her boss seemed to ignore her needs as an employee. She did not have a regular computer to use, and as half of her working time she was required to input data, she found that this impacted on her work. Constantly 'hovering' near her colleagues' desks, in order to find a computer she could use, affected her relationships with them negatively.

For months she tried to broach the subject with her boss. She tried to do this subtly and indirectly. On the way to the coffee room she tentatively mentioned to him, 'There's most likely nothing you can do but it would be nice for me to have a computer I could use regularly. I do know that space is cramped and other people have priority.' Sarah desperately wanted her boss to pick up on what she was trying to say but instead he simply responded, 'Yeah, it's a bit cramped, the building's not good,' as he left the room.

Similar conversations occurred for several months. When she mentioned to her partner what was going on at work he became angry and responded, 'You should just go and tell him, it's not good enough ... they're taking the mick out of you.' Sarah had mixed feelings about this. On the one hand her partner had validated that it was unacceptable for her not to have a computer for her sole use and she felt 'fired up' enough to go in and say something, but on the other hand it made her feel like a wimp that she had not been able to sort it out to date. Eventually, in order to shut her partner up, she took it up with her boss again.

With a tremor in her voice she asked, 'May I have a word with you?' After there was no response she raised her voice slightly. 'John, I need to speak to you.' Her boss turned round. 'I need a computer I can use whenever I choose. You obviously don't take me seriously enough to give me one, and that makes me feel rubbish. Everyone I have spoken to thinks it's out of order that I haven't got one.'

As you can imagine, this was met with a defensive response from John who asked what side of the bed Sarah had got out of, locating the problem firmly in her court. A heated discussion followed, resulting in Sarah being pulled up about her bad attitude.

If only Sarah had known about the assertiveness strategies that she later learnt. It was too late for that job but the methods she subsequently learnt held her in good stead in subsequent workplaces.

Expressing Your Feelings, Needs and Points of View

Sometimes the way we let people know our views or how we feel seems to increase the likelihood of our receiving a negative outcome, such as not being taken seriously or provoking an argument. We may be too passive/submissive or too aggressive in our approach to others, to the same disappointing effect. It is therefore helpful to work out ways in which we can express our feelings, needs and points of view in an assertive manner.

The following two formulas can prove very helpful to this end.

*I think/feel/need*_____ *This is based on*_____

_____

_____

_____

I think it would be helpful if _____

_____

_____

_____

Can we discuss this?

Alternatively:

When you do/say _____ *I feel* _____

_____

_____

_____

_____*and I would prefer* _____

_____

_____

_____

Can we discuss this?

As you can see, the first approach addresses your own needs, feelings or thoughts first and then the explanation follows, while the second turns this around and puts the other person's actions or words first, with your feelings being expressed afterwards. This illustrates there is no right or wrong way to approach assertiveness. What is important is to find something that works for you and seems to 'map on to' how you may say something naturally.

Finishing with the question 'Can we discuss this?' acknowledges that the other person may have important thoughts and feelings about this that you are maybe not aware of and it may help to discuss these.

The following are examples of how these formulas might work in practice:

I think I am not being taken seriously at work *because* none of the ideas I come up with in meetings is ever acted upon. *I think it would be helpful if* you could give me feedback after meetings about any ideas I have expressed so that I can understand why they may not be viable. *Can we discuss this?*

When you leave the house in a mess *I feel* as though you don't care about me and just expect me to clean up after you. *I would prefer it* if you tidied up after yourself or tell me why this is difficult for you so I can understand it better.

I need to have some time to myself every so often. *This is because* I get stressed when life is so busy. *I would like* a little bit of free time as it would make me happier, more relaxed and would make me feel cared for by you. I am not sure what you think. *Can we discuss this?*

As you can see from the examples given above, there is a range of ways you can use this assertiveness strategy. It's OK for you to amend, as you see fit, the exact wording. For example, it may be that you replace 'based on' with 'because', or 'I would prefer' with 'I would like' as different terms may seem more natural to you.

When you say 'I feel' it leaves less opportunity for people to disagree with you. This is in stark contrast to statements such as 'You make me . . .', 'You're out of order', 'You are winding me up', which are more likely to trigger disagreement. As such, these assertive ways of expressing ourselves are often called 'I' statements, in contrast to 'you' statements.

These new ways of expressing yourself may seem difficult to remember, especially in situations where you feel strong emotions such as anger, or anxiety, but the more you practise them, the more naturally they will come to mind. Practising may involve writing down what you want to say or saying it out loud when you are on your own. It may involve practising in front of other people who have your best interests at heart and can give you constructive feedback. Some people find practising in front of a mirror very helpful. Most of all *having a go*, maybe initially in easier situations and building up to more difficult ones, can help you hone this way of expressing yourself so that eventually it begins to 'roll off your tongue' quite naturally. Worksheet 8 in Chapter 12 may be of use to help you break things down into clear and manageable steps.

Once you have practised what you want to say, a further component of the exercise, one with which you will be very familiar by now, is to evoke a supportive frame of mind to help you say what you want to say. Self-assertiveness may be anxiety-provoking, at least until it becomes a regular part of your life. So, before you approach the person with whom you wish to assert yourself, engage in your soothing rhythm breathing for a minute or so. When you are ready, bring to mind your chosen compassionate image or evoke the sense of your ideal compassionate self. Remind yourself of the key compassionate qualities. Feel a sense of warmth and calm together with strength and courage. Adjust your posture, feeling strength in your spine and openness and warmth in your facial expression. Now approach the person and say what you have been planning and practising to say.

Using a 'hook' to motivate others to change their behaviour

Unfortunately, despite our best efforts, other people may not change their behaviour. This may be because they can't or they find it difficult. However, it may be because they are not able to empathize with your situation or because they need to see what's in it for them. If you find yourself in this situation it may be helpful to add a 'hook' to the exercise. In other words, tell them what's in it for them. For example, a change in their behaviour may mean you are less anxious and therefore you would be easier to be around, it may build your self-confidence so you can take on more roles at work or it may mean that you feel more valued and therefore seek reassurance from them less.

Exercise 52: Communicating how we feel and what our needs are

Now it's time for you to have a go:

Step 1: Bring to mind a situation where you were having difficulty expressing yourself.

Step 2: Using the examples on pages 224–225 for a guide, work out what you want to say and how you can say it.

Step 3: Plan when you are going to speak to the person.

Step 4: Practise – be it on your own, with someone you trust, or in front of the mirror.

Step 5: Make use of exercises you have found helpful in the past. For example, use the compassionate behavioural experiment worksheet on page 210 to help you prepare to implement your plan, or write a compassionate letter to yourself, or sit in the presence of your compassionate coach and gain strength and encouragement from them.

Step 6: Express yourself to the person in question.

Step 7: Review how it went using the worksheet on page 215 (used previously to review your compassionate behavioural experiment), write a compassionate letter to yourself with respect to this exercise or use imagery – especially if things did not go quite as you had hoped.

Reflection on Exercise 52

There will be situations that you cannot plan for or be *proactive* about. Situations may require you to be *reactive*; you may be put on the spot and need to say something quickly. In such situations it is helpful to take a soothing breath then feel strength in your spine and, if you can, bring to mind the above ways of expressing yourself in an assertive manner. The more you do this, the more naturally they will come to you.

Unfortunately, many of us find that the changes we are trying to make are often resisted by others. People get used to us being a particular way and interact with us accordingly. This can be very frustrating. If you find this is the case for you it may be worth addressing the issue directly.

Linda's story

When Linda attempted the assertiveness exercise on pages 226–227 at work things generally went the way she had hoped. However, when she tried it in relation to her partner, he simply responded: 'Have you been reading some of that self-help again?' In addition one of her sisters just shrugged her shoulders and said she did not have the time to discuss things. Linda therefore thought long and hard about this and finally responded to her partner: 'When you say things like that to me it hurts because I feel as though you don't want me to be more self-confident. I am trying my best. It would be great if you could help me with this because I think it would be good for me and for our relationship. Can we discuss this?'

With her sister she felt as though she could not take another direct snub again so instead she emailed her, saying: 'I know you said you did not have time to discuss things with me, but this only makes me feel more sure that you don't value me as a friend and sister. It would be good if you could spare some time to talk, but if you can't that is OK as well – at least I can say that I have tried.'

Both strategies resulted in good outcomes. With her partner the first conversation itself brought them closer together. He started to take an interest in the changes Linda was trying to make and, in addition, changed his own behaviour towards her. He even started to use this way of expressing himself at home and at work.

With Linda's sister nothing changed. She did not even respond to the email, but Linda felt proud that she had stood her ground in this way. She reassured herself every so often by thinking, 'This is about her, not me. I have tried but I'm not going to bang my head against a brick wall.'

Exercise 53: Giving constructive feedback

Most of us fear upsetting other people and this can prevent us from giving constructive feedback, which may result in our avoiding an issue entirely or skirting round it. It can also lead to frustration with other people (and with ourselves) as patterns of behaviour go on repeating themselves.

Although the previous exercise may be helpful in such situations, other relationships require us to be less focused on our own needs, feelings and views and more receptive to the needs of someone else or, at work, an organization or company.

If you find giving constructive feedback difficult, work through the steps below and see if this is helpful to you. Isaac's story (page 230) illustrates this process further.

Step 1: Think about the person to whom you wish to give some constructive feedback and bring to mind the specific issue you wish to deal with.

Step 2: Take a few breaths and bring to mind a compassionate image or the ideal compassionate self; remind yourself of the key compassionate qualities – strength and courage but, importantly here, empathy and non-judgement also.

Step 3: Remind yourself that you wish the other person to be the best that they can be. You wish to help their development.

Step 4: Now think what the person in question needs to know, employing the following formula: '*I want you to know that............It is important that I tell you this because............Can we discuss this?*

Step 5: Now plan how and when you are going to give your feedback.

Step 6: Practise – be it on your own, with someone you trust or in front of the mirror.

Step 7: Make use of exercises you have found helpful in the past. For example, use the compassionate behavioural experiment worksheet on page 210 to help prepare you for implementing your plan. This is likely to include what you are going to do in the moments before you speak to the person in question, write a compassionate letter to yourself, sit in the presence of your compassionate coach and gain strength and encouragement from them.

Step 8: Express yourself to the person in question.

Step 9: Review how it went using worksheet 9 on page 215. Write a compassionate letter to yourself with respect to this exercise or use imagery – especially if things did not go quite as you had hoped.

Isaac's story

Isaac found that one of the new members of his team, Andrew, regularly arrived late for work. At first he ignored it, thinking his colleague must have had problems predicting the traffic or the buses, and reassured himself that eventually things would sort themselves out. But as time went on the problem continued. Isaac started hovering round reception at the time that Andrew usually arrived and looking at the clock as he approached the office, but this did not seem to have any effect at all. Isaac became increasingly angry with Andrew, thinking, 'You're taking the mick', while also being annoyed with himself, thinking: 'Stand up for yourself', 'You're pathetic'. Isaac found that he was short with Andrew when he had dealings with him, tended to look at his work with a more critical eye than was warranted, and even got to the point where he could not be around the other man in the canteen or coffee room without his blood boiling.

This was clearly not a good situation for Isaac, Andrew, or the rest of the team. They could see someone getting away with bad time-keeping, felt resentful themselves and were aware of tension in the work environment.

In this situation Andrew could have used the strategy outlined in Exercise 52 above but it seemed inappropriate to be talking about his own needs, feelings and thoughts in this situation. Instead he decided it would be beneficial to give Andrew some constructive feedback instead. That evening he used imagery to remind himself of the key compassionate qualities, especially courage, empathy and non-judgement, and thought about Andrew from this perspective. 'I want him to be the best that he can be,' thought Isaac.

He imagined himself saying to Andrew, 'I want you to know that the working day starts at 9 a.m. and yet I have noticed that you regularly arrive later than that. It is important that we discuss this because it has an impact on the work you do, the rest of the team, and also on you as well. Can we discuss it?'

Once Isaac had imagined himself saying this he realized that it might be best to have the discussion away from the main part of the office and potential interruptions, allowing space and time for it. He ran through what he was going to say a few times, and used compassionate imagery and soothing rhythm breathing to recruit the appropriate frame of mind, one that would be non-judgemental, warm, empathic and strong. The night before he planned to have the discussion, Isaac used the compassionate behavioural experiment worksheet (page 210) to help him think through what he was about to do and also wrote a letter to himself in his journal.

The next day Isaac carefully followed his plan. He engaged in his breathing exercise, reminded himself of the key compassionate qualities and, with warmth in his face and voice, asked to speak to Andrew. After he had said what he had to say he calmly waited for a response. Andrew paused. It seemed that the air of calm that Isaac had adopted had rubbed off on him and he sat quietly for a few moments. He then responded, 'Yes, I know I am terrible at time-keeping and usually late. All I can say is I am sorry and I will make a concerted effort from here on in.' After a discussion of the practicalities of him getting in on time and how his time-keeping would be reviewed, Andrew got up to leave and on the way out stated, 'Thanks for being so good about it, I will do better.'

Reflection on Exercise 53

As with the previous exercise, further preparation for taking action may involve you working through some of the strategies you have tried before, such as compassionate alternative thoughts/images, writing a compassionate letter to yourself and/or using the compassionate behavioural experiment worksheet. By now you will know what other ancillary exercises may be helpful to you to supplement this exercise.

Remember that if you are giving constructive feedback from this mindset, you are doing it with the other person's best interests at heart – just like the compassionate teacher in Chapter 3. Their role was to nurture those around them to be the best they could be, which involved giving feedback without judgement. So, turning the focus from ourselves to what the other person needs to grow and be 'at their best' can give us the strength and courage to act. It obviously has a huge impact on our own self-confidence also.

Making Seemingly Small Behavioural Changes

Although this book has focused on increasing your self-confidence, now that it is hopefully building it is worth seeing if small behavioural changes also, maybe in the areas of your life you feel confident in as well as areas in which you feel less so, can have a positive effect on your own happiness and that of others. This can further develop your self-confidence, directly or indirectly.

If you decide to make some of the changes suggested in the box on page 234 it may be beneficial to explore the following guidance:

1. Make sure you 'mix it up'

Engage in a range of new behaviours over time rather than picking only one or two and sticking to them. Research tells us that we 'habituate' or quickly get used to the positive benefits of any activity over time. For example, you may really appreciate a new plant you have bought for a room but, after a week or two, it is likely that you come to take it for granted and gain less pleasure from seeing it. Similarly you may get a buzz from having a positive encounter with someone for the first time, but ten such meetings later it may feel less rewarding.

2. Incorporate changes into your daily life

One study split a number of students into two groups. Group A were instructed to do five 'random acts of kindness' all *in one day* while group B were told to do one random act of kindness *per day* over five days. Group B were found to be significantly happier at the end of the experiment even though they had done the same amount of 'acts' – if you combine this practice with 'mixing up' your other activities it is a very significant step towards becoming a happier you.

Although the studies above were looking at happiness per se, I would suggest that those whose level of happiness is increased are likely to feel more self-confident as a result.

Andy's story

Andy, whom we first met in Chapter 4, had slowly and methodically worked through all the stages of the Compassionate Mind approach to building his self-confidence and had developed a toolkit of practices and strategies that he found helpful to him. He was surprised that he had found the strength to tackle a number of difficult things both at work and in his personal life and felt as though his main focus should be on practising certain mindfulness and imagery exercises (self-practice) to maintain and strengthen the gains he had made. Andy recognized that in relation to the three circle diagram (Diagram 1, Chapter 2) much of this work was directed at developing self-compassion further in order to regulate his still sensitive threat system.

Andy did, however, feel an urge to see how else he could consciously change his life in the pursuit of more enjoyment. He reflected that, to date, he had avoided so many things in the past due to his lack of self-confidence. He felt that in the past his 'drive system' was caught up with trying to prove himself and keeping his mind away from thinking about his past but now it was motivating him towards experimenting in potentially positive ways. Andy therefore reviewed the list in the box on page 234 and started to put entries into his diary to remind him to do certain things. Entries included 'random act of kindness day', 'karaoke night', 'new situation day', 'funny film night' and 'hello to five people in the street day'. He reflected that he would find some of these things relatively easy whilst others filled him with dread. As such, some days he achieved his goal without much preparation whilst others took a considerable amount of preparation to make sure they happened. Two weeks later, Andy reflected that he felt positive, in both a drive/achievement way but also because he had continued his self-practice, content within himself and around other people. Some of the exercises had built his self-confidence directly whilst others, he reflected, seemed to be working indirectly.

Here are a few ideas that people have previously found beneficial:

Sign up to a campaign or volunteer for something you believe in.

Make some changes to your home environment. This may involve buying a plant or some flowers, putting a photo up that reminds you of good times or important relationships, tidying up the house or your garden.

Engage in brief opportunities for mindfulness such as mindful hand washing, stretching or drinking.

At certain points in the day, or triggered by certain events, encourage yourself to stop, drop your shoulders, take a soothing breath.

Go for a walk and smile or say hello to someone as you walk down the street – if you can only manage a fleeting smile at first, try gradually to increase this to holding the other person's gaze for slightly longer next time.

When you pay at the till for your shopping, make sure you make some eye contact and small talk with the cashier.

Watch a film that makes you laugh or gives you a sense of warmth.

Experiment with new situations – just to see what happens.

Make an effort to help someone in your neighbourhood who is in need of it.

Take some things that you no longer need to the charity shop and savour the act of giving.

Engage in a 'random act of kindness', maybe to someone you know, maybe to a stranger – this can range from a kind word to a warm gesture.

Do something that you used to enjoy doing. This does not have to be something you have enjoyed as an adult – it may be something you enjoyed as a child, such as going to a fair, sitting on a beach, drawing, sewing or maintaining your bike.

Have a look around and see whether you can draw inspiration from other people – how are they spending their time?

Exercise 54: Making seemingly small changes

Now it's your turn!

Step 1: Put together your own list of things you think it would be good to do.

Step 2: Allocate tasks to specific days of the week.

Step 3: Prepare for the activities using the ways suggested in previous chapters.

Step 4: Engage in the activities.

Step 5: If it is helpful, review how you have got on in your notebook or journal, or by using the compassionate behavioural experiment reflections sheet (page 215).

Reflection on Exercise 54

Making these small behavioural changes can be a very positive and uplifting experience, but take care to maintain and further develop your contentment and soothing system at the same time. Remember, our drive system is powerful and can give us a real buzz and sense of achievement. But you need to keep all three systems in balance – working on one to the detriment or neglect of another can lead to coming 'unstuck' when things maybe don't go quite to plan. It is self-compassion that will support you through the difficult times as well as helping you build resilience towards life's inevitable knocks and setbacks.

Savouring Positive Experiences

Life can be so busy that it is all too easy to spend the majority of our time thinking about what we have got to do next, or what we have just done, instead of appreciating the present moment.

Consciously *savouring* our positive experiences can enhance their emotional impact. It can also help create a more vivid memory store on which we can draw at a later date, turning a conscious moment of contentment or happiness into many more. It is a very simple strategy that involves stopping and appreciating a particular point in time. You could savour the sense of achievement you get when you have successfully faced a difficult situation, a moment of exhilaration, a moment of clarity, a moment of awe when you appreciate some beautiful scenery, for instance, or a moment when you feel really connected to those around you. You may also choose to savour the experience of being in freshly changed bed linen, having a welcome hot drink, stepping inside a warm house and closing the door on a wintry evening, or stretching when you have got up after a restful night's sleep.

Because the exercises you are completing throughout this book are aimed at building your self-confidence, it may perhaps be a good thing to concentrate on savouring these experiences in particular. For instance, the sense of achievement you get after you have engaged in a compassionate behavioural experiment or the positive feedback you receive when something has gone well. But, of course, it may equally be helpful to you to savour a whole range of situations – big and small. Whatever works best for you is OK.

Exercise 55: Savouring positive experiences

Step 1: Notice a positive experience or stop to appreciate a moment in time – no matter how small.

Step 2: Take a soothing breath and relax your shoulders.

Step 3: Appreciate the moment.

Step 4: Work through your senses – what can you see, what can you hear, what can you smell, feel, taste? Linger on each of these sensations in turn.

Step 5: When you are ready, take another soothing breath and return your attention to your surroundings.

Reflection on Exercise 55

Savouring is similar to mindfulness, in that it encourages you to be 'in the moment'. However, while mindfulness focuses more on *observing*, or at least this was the way it was used in Chapter 7, savouring involves *appreciating* moments in time and experiencing a sense of warmth while doing so.

Many people find that they can strengthen the positive effects of savouring by regularly recording in their journal or diary particular moments that they have savoured. It can also help to recall positive experiences, especially when we are feeling low or anxious, as they can help lift our mood. Some people find that taking a photograph of something they are savouring will act to boost their mood, both at the time and in the future – this is why so many of us tend to have photos around to 'capture' and remind us of particular experiences. But remember, it would be a good idea to savour a whole *range* of experiences and to change the display of photos in which you recorded them from time to time as they can lose their power otherwise.

Acceptance

In life there are things that we can change and adjust and things that, no matter how hard we try, we are unable to do anything about. It is likely that you have become more aware of this while working your way through this book. For example, you may have surprised yourself by now being able to do certain things that you previously felt were impossible for you. However, this may be accompanied by a feeling of sadness that you were unable to do such things in the past. In addition you may be aware that things such as your fundamental appearance or certain aspects of your personality are also difficult, if not impossible, to change.

The concept – and, more importantly, the *feeling* – of acceptance can help us come to terms with such things. Acceptance is not about being defeated. Instead it can be a very powerful state of mind, a strong foundation upon which to base new developments in our lives.

Although it is useful to develop acceptance of the things we cannot change, it can also be helpful to develop acceptance of how things are for you at present. The exercise overleaf therefore asks you to focus on this moment in time.

The 'perfect' illusion

One of the reasons why people suffer with poor self-confidence is because they try – and fail – to be perfect. When they don't achieve what they set out to do, they give themselves a hard time. If you think this may be the case for you too, ask yourself the following question: Would you like someone who was *perfect?*

I personally find it difficult to be around people whom I perceive as perfect. I can easily be intimidated by them, and as a consequence I don't tend to feel good about myself while I'm around them.

If I think back to times in my life when an acquaintance has become a friend, it has usually come about when something has happened to make them seem like a human being who is *not* perfect. For example, when 'perfect' Sarah let me know that she was struggling with work and was worried about it, things between us changed. She turned from being someone with whom I engaged in social chit-chat to someone with whom I had a connection. Her admission made me see her as a human being. I felt flattered that she had confided in me. It gave me an opportunity to feel I was of help to her, and our friendship developed from that point.

To drive this message home further, in the film *Good Will Hunting*, Robin Williams's character defends his late wife by passionately stating that it was her *idiosyncrasies* and *imperfections* that made her perfect in his eyes. Watch the film if you haven't seen it. Or, if you have, watch it again, because the message is delivered very powerfully. This is something I bring to mind whenever I find that self-criticism has been triggered in me by viewing myself, or my actions, as 'imperfect'. It helps me be self-compassionate and ultimately to accept myself, idiosyncrasies (and, boy, there are a lot of them!) and all.

Close consideration of things we cannot change can be emotionally draining. It may be helpful for you initially to work on things that are likely to produce *relatively* less powerful emotions. As you become more practised in this way of working, you can move on to the things that are more challenging for you. And read Marie's story, on page 240, for an example of how this exercise helped someone accept problems with their appearance and achieve more self-confidence as a result.

Exercise 56: Accepting yourself and things that you cannot change

As you have done with many of the previous exercises, find a place you can be relatively undisturbed for 10–15 minutes or so. A place that is free from distractions, and where you feel comfortable to engage in an imagery exercise. Sit with strength in your spine, and with feelings of openness and warmth. Bring a slight smile to your face.

Step 1: Bring to mind something that you wish you could change but cannot. You may choose something that happened in the past or something in the present.

Step 2: Engage with your soothing rhythm breathing and, when you are ready, bring to mind your ideal compassionate self or a compassionate image. This may be your perfect nurturer, compassionate coach or compassionate companion.

Step 3: Remind yourself of the key qualities of compassion, experiencing each of them in turn.

Step 4: Now bring your attention to the aspect of your life that you cannot change. Invite your ideal compassionate self or compassionate image to recognize the disappointment you feel that change is not possible.

Step 5: Now think about what the ideal compassionate self or compassionate image might say about this…………how would their voice sound?…………What emotions would they be directing towards you? …………….Are there colours……………smells……………sounds associated with this experience?...............Consider this for a few minutes.

Step 6: If possible experience a sensation of peace. A sense of calm, a sense of acceptance ....once again allowing this to last for a while.

Step 7: When you are ready, return to your soothing rhythm breathing and let the image and the experience fade from your mind, slowly bringing your awareness back to your surroundings.

Marie's story

When Marie looked at these exercises she was immediately aware of a number of things she wished to address. She had lost her mum to cancer when she was only three years old and had later suffered at the hands of her step-mum. She was bullied at school and had had a couple of difficult relationships – it seemed as though her life after three years old could be represented by a line of dominoes falling down one after another. The diagrammatic formulation and imagery exercises had helped her grieve and feel less anger about a number of things but she felt she still had work to do.

Marie also identified that there were things in the here and now that she wanted to change but couldn't. She was self-conscious about her appearance, more specifically her crooked smile and large nose. When she managed to ask people she cared about for feedback on this, they reacted kindly but confirmed that she did indeed have a crooked smile and a large nose. Despite this she felt OK in their company, knowing they would love her whatever, but with others she felt extremely self-conscious and would bow her head, avoid smiling and, sometimes, avoid social situations altogether.

Marie had found compassionate behavioural experiments very useful but still felt that she was struggling to accept her looks. She decided to work further on acceptance of her appearance. During the exercise she brought to mind how she looked and imagined sitting in the presence of her compassionate coach. She imagined her compassionate coach extending their arms and holding her face between their hands. She heard them softly say: 'You are who you are............you are OK ....there is no need to hang your head............feel the strength to hold your head up high ....when things are difficult take a breath ....feel the warmth, the strength and courage............face the world.'

This exercise changed Marie's life dramatically. Although it brought her to tears at the time, she felt the strength and courage she needed to face the world in a spirit of self-acceptance. The other experiments she engaged in suddenly seemed easier to do, setbacks were easier to recover from and her self-confidence grew.

Reflection on Exercise 56

As in the case of previous exercises, especially those using imagery, you may find that your self-critic attempts to undermine your efforts. If this is the case, remind them that you are both on the same team and there are alternative and more helpful ways, other than self-criticism, for you to achieve your goals.

As previously stated, it can be difficult to undertake these exercises so it may be helpful for you to plan to do something for yourself as a reward after you have been working on them. Have a warm bath, go for a walk, see a friend, put some uplifting music on or, if it helps, have a sleep.

Exercise 57: Embracing who you are

In contrast to the previous exercise, which is often associated with a sense of gentleness and warmth, people often find this one to be energizing. Of course, both exercises aim to help you feel a sense of inner strength.

Once again, start with something that is relatively easy for you and move on to things that are more difficult later.

Find a place where you can be undisturbed for 10–15 minutes or so, one that is free from distractions and where you can comfortably engage in an imagery exercise.

Step 1: Bring to mind something that is associated with difficult feelings for you. Something that you cannot change and have difficulty accepting. It may be an aspect of your appearance, part of your personality, something that has happened to you or something that is going on at the moment.

Step 2: Now stand up. Feel strength and alertness in your spine. Engage in your soothing rhythm breathing. With each breath feel your chest expand. Adjust your posture to evoke strength.

Step 3: If it helps, inhabit your ideal compassionate self. Alternatively imagine your compassionate image standing with you, maybe behind you, maybe alongside, with their hand on your shoulder.

Step 4: Now, with both warmth and strength, make a statement such as the following: *I am a human being who has amazing capacities and abilities. It is normal for me to struggle in certain areas, and at certain times. I am human ....I am not perfect............I have/am/have experienced............It is understandable for me to have difficulty with this............But I am resilient and I can accept this about myself.*

Stay with this feeling for a while.

Step 5: When you are ready, return to your soothing rhythm breathing. Once more feel a sense of strength and alertness in your posture and your mind. Now let the experience fade, slowly bringing your awareness back to your surroundings.

Reflection on Exercise 57

During many of these exercises it is most beneficial to experience a balance of all of the key qualities of compassion. However, in this exercise it can be more helpful to focus on specific components of it, primarily strength and courage.

Here are a few statements that people have previously found it helpful to use during this exercise:

At this moment in time I am not as self-confident as I would like to be.

I am a survivor.

I have survived difficult things.

I am a shy person.

I have a stammer.

I have a big nose – so what?

During the exercise the aim is not to feel apologetic but rather to feel strength and a sense of self-confidence, even with respect to something you usually find it difficult to accept. Your compassionate image may help you with this.

Adjusting your posture during the exercise, until you feel a sense of strength and self-confidence, can also be extremely helpful.

Exercise 58: Accepting your situation, right here, right now

This exercise is similar to the previous one, but instead of focusing on something that you cannot change, or something you are unlikely to be able to change, the focus is on accepting where you find yourself right now.

Find a place you can be relatively undisturbed for 10–15 minutes or so. A place that is free from distractions, where you feel comfortable to engage in an imagery exercise.

Step 1: While standing up, feel strength in your spine and a sense of alertness. Engage in your soothing rhythm breathing. With each breath, feel your chest expand and, if it helps, adjust your posture to evoke a sense of strength.

Step 2: If it helps, imagine your ideal compassionate self or other compassionate image standing with you, maybe behind you, maybe alongside, with their hand on your shoulder.

Step 3: Now, with both warmth and strength, make a statement such as the following:

I am a human being who has amazing capacities and abilities ....it is normal for me to struggle in certain areas, and at certain times – I am human... ....I am not perfect but I can accept myself for who I am right in this moment.

Stay with this experience for a few moments.

Step 4: When you are ready, return to your soothing rhythm breathing. Once more feel a sense of strength and alertness in your posture and your mind. Now let the experience fade, slowly bringing your awareness back to where you are standing.

Reflection on Exercise 58

For many people written preparation for exercises 57 and 58 can be helpful. Allowing yourself the time to create a statement that is both meaningful and personal to you can help to enhance your self-confidence as well as helping you to carry out this exercise to the best effect.

Although some people find it easy to voice a statement such as the one above out loud, others prefer to speak the words in their mind. If this is the case for you, I would encourage you to build up gradually to speaking the words aloud. Time and time again, people report that saying as well as hearing the words has more of an impact on them.

Tone of voice and rate of speech, as well as posture, are key. Play around with the exercise in order to increase its benefit to you. Once again, you may need to work up to a confidently delivered statement, first starting in a whisper and slowly building upon this. Rate of speech is important too as you need to take time to *feel* what you are saying, allowing the limbic system to register it.

Finally, it can be helpful to engage in this exercise in front of those you trust and care about. If you are able to do this, make sure that you engage in some degree of eye contact as visual feedback from others can be very important.

Using Self-compassion to Guide Your Day

It is hoped that during your reading of this book you have tried all manner of compassionate exercises aimed at building your self-confidence. Hopefully some of these will become part of your personal daily or weekly practice. Here is a penultimate, very brief yet powerful exercise. It is one that I personally use all the time.

I find that when I feel anxious about certain things at work, avoidance strikes. For example, I hate making phone calls that *may* be awkward and so I will find all manner of excuses to avoid picking up the phone. When I eventually make the call I feel an incredible sense of relief. I wonder why on earth I had been avoiding the task and swear that I won't do it again. Despite this, guess what happens the following week?

Well, without my self-compassionate practice, this pattern would repeat itself over and over again. I am not saying I never avoid such things now, but on the days I practise this exercise I tend to do what I need to do – I feel better about my work, happier with myself, and molehills don't end up becoming mountains.

Exercise 59: Guiding your day with self-compassion

Step 1: Take a soothing breath, calm your mind and your body.

Step 2: Bring to mind your ideal compassionate self or a compassionate image.

Step 3: Now, slowly and warmly, ask your ideal compassionate self or compassionate image the following question:

What can I do for myself today that will make tomorrow a better day?

Step 4: Imagine how you will feel if you manage to do the thing or things you brought to mind in Step 3.

Step 5: Take a soothing breath, feel a sense of strength and warmth.

Step 6: Now be guided by your own compassionate advice.

Using Self-compassion to Help You *In* Difficult Situations

I don't know about you but when I find myself in a situation where my self-confidence is low or feeling dented, I tend to question myself *a lot*. I not only question what I have done, but also what it would be beneficial to do now to make myself feel better. Sometimes this results in my mind seemingly 'shutting down'; at other times it seems to 'blow a fuse'. My anxious brain tells me one thing, my upset brain tells me something else, and my angry brain contradicts both – seemingly simultaneously.

Many of the exercises outlined above have been introduced with the explicit instruction that you should start with something easy, finding a place where you feel comfortable and taking a certain amount of time for reflection. It is hoped that, as time goes by, such practices will 'train your brain' so that different frames of mind become more readily accessible and an integral part of your life.

However, what can help you *during* situations you find yourself in *now*? This final exercise is an abbreviated version of previous exercises, to help guide you *in the moment*. That is not to say that this practice guarantees that you will make the right decision or do the right thing at any point in time, but it can help. I find it invaluable.

Exercise 60 : Using self-compassion in difficult situations

When you find yourself in the middle of a difficult situation:

Step 1: Take a soothing breath.

Step 2: Alter your posture and maybe your facial expression in a way that will evoke a sense of compassion and a sense of calmness and strength.

Step 3: Take a moment.

Step 4: Now let this 'frame of mind' guide you.

Reflection on Exercise 60

This exercise is aimed at altering your frame of mind *in* situations, with the aim of altering the way you feel, the thoughts that you have, what you attend to and what action, or inaction, you take. You are consciously stepping out of your threat system and into a compassionate mindset.

Personally, I notice that when engaging in this practice, if I am standing I tend to take a step to one side as a change in position helps me to change my perspective. If I am sitting I also adjust my posture, maybe shifting my weight on my seat, changing the crossing of my legs or simply adjusting my back against the upright of the chair. As you have hopefully experienced, small postural changes can have a significant impact.

Compassionate imagery or the ideal compassionate self are not the only ways of changing your frame of mind quickly. Some people have described how imagining a particular colour can help them, while others have found the use of a familiar scent, on a tissue or handkerchief, to be a quick and beneficial way for them to gain a clearer perspective on a situation and regain their self-confidence. You may have found some of these strategies helpful while practising previous exercises in this book and, if this is the case, it may be useful to adopt them in conjunction with this exercise.

Conclusions

In this chapter we have looked at a number of different strategies to help you build your self-confidence. In the final chapter we will translate what you have found helpful so far into a regular form of practice to equip you for your onward journey.

14 Reflections and Future Directions

In the early chapters of this book we discussed how self-confidence is something we build and maintain, rather than something we either have or haven't got. It is hoped that this new understanding will help counteract some of the shame and self-criticism you may previously have experienced in relation to low self-confidence. In addition, thinking about self-confidence in this way will hopefully help you to develop a sense that things *can* change.

We then went on to look at the evolutionary origins of self-confidence, how and why we often undermine ourselves, and how developing self-compassion can help. Understanding ourselves can be a further key to 'letting go' of our self-criticism and shame, and directing us towards more fertile ground on which we can build our self-confidence. This is why we spent some time looking at the way our biological make-up and life experiences can affect us, the ways we then learn to cope with life and the unintended drawbacks and consequences we often encounter.

We then explored what compassion is and how the views we have of ourselves can stop us developing it. We reflected that contrary to the popular view that it is the 'easy option', 'wishy-washy' or involves 'letting ourselves off the hook', the development of self-compassion can be a difficult path to tread, one that requires strength and courage. It involves us confronting our past, our present and our future, and all that they bring with them.

We prepared for the development or enhancement of compassion with a number of exercises. We discussed various ways of practising mindfulness. We then went on to practise soothing rhythm breathing and finding a place of contentment. We used compassionate imagery in a number of ways, ranging from exploring how compassion feels in the mind and body, to embodying the ideal compassionate self and developing a compassionate coach, companion, teacher or nurturer.

Finally, compassionate thinking, letter writing and behaviours, as well as a number of other exercises such as those involving assertiveness, were introduced as a means for you to address your self-criticism and feelings of shame, and ultimately find ways to further build your self-confidence.

In this chapter we will now focus on two final areas:

- Looking at your life as a story of strength and resilience
- Developing a template for self-practice that will build your self-confidence further

It is hoped that these two things will help you develop a more balanced view of yourself and give you a plan for the future.

Looking at Your Life as a Story of Strength and Resilience

Throughout this book we have reflected on the amazing capacities we human beings possess. We have looked at the way in which a combination of influences and experiences leads us to adopt certain ways of thinking, feeling and behaving. When circumstances lead us to struggle with our self-confidence we can become more prone to avoid things, adopt a social 'mask' with others, or constantly strive in vain for perfection, engage in self-criticism and experience high levels of anxiety and shame.

I hope that the formulation exercise in Chapter 4 allowed you to gain a greater understanding of how past experiences might have affected you, and what you tend to do in order to cope with this. However, because

Exercise 8 was focused on understanding your difficulties, it is quite likely that the formulation you developed failed to recognize your resilience, strength and *positive* attributes. The following exercise is therefore designed to redress the balance.

Exercise 61: Updating your formulation

Before you begin, have the formulation you developed in Chapter 4 to hand. It also may help you to read Andy's updated story and formulation to give you a clear idea of what this exercise is asking you to do.

Find a place that is, as far as possible, free from distractions. Somewhere you can be for 10–15 minutes. Sit in a relaxed, open posture that has *strength* or *alertness* in it. It is a good idea to close your eyes for the start of this exercise but you may prefer to lower your gaze instead and settle it on a low fixed point.

If it is helpful to you, start by using your soothing rhythm breathing or place of contentment image. Alternatively use one of the mindfulness practices from pages 103–13. After some minutes practise your preferred compassionate imagery exercise. This may be your ideal compassionate self, compassionate coach/teacher/companion/nurturer. With the help of this image, evoke your compassionate mindset, reminding yourself of all the key qualities this brings with it.

When you are ready, review the 'influences and experiences' part of your formulation (the first box on the left of the page). Take a few soothing breaths as you review the information held there. Now, with the warmth of the compassionate mind, slowly ask yourself the following questions, allowing yourself time to think and reflect on each one:

• Given that I have coped with these things, what can I compassionately conclude about myself?

• How can I view my strengths and qualities?

- Although such influences and experiences have resulted in difficulties, are there any positives that have come out of them? For example, people who have been through difficulties themselves are often more sensitive to the needs of others.

If you have been able to come up with some compassionate views or conclusions about yourself, draw a new box maybe underneath the 'key concerns and fears' one. Now draw a strong arrow from the 'influences and experiences' box towards it. Write the heading 'key strengths and qualities' in the new box. Next, write into it the compassionate conclusions you have drawn above.

Once you have done this, take a soothing breath and return to the questions again – allowing time for further compassionate conclusions to be drawn.

Return to your soothing rhythm breathing, feeling a sense of things slowing down. Now, with warmth, slowly read each of the 'key strengths and qualities' you have written. Consider each in turn. Allow them to 'sink in'.

Andy's updated story

We met Andy in Chapters 4 and 11, whilst looking at formulations and compassionate letter writing. His experiences and feelings were charted in his original formulation (see page 61). But as time passed Andy began to recognize that the diagram he had worked on so diligently only seemed to give one side of his life story. He therefore set about redressing this imbalance. Reviewing the notes and letters he had written in his journal, and looking at the questions provided in exercise 61, he began drawing ideas together relating to his resilience, strength and *positive* attributes. Andy then used this information to update his formulation (Diagram 6, page 255).

Once the exercise was completed, Andy took a few soothing breaths and read it through. As he did so he felt his self-confidence building further. Andy was so positive about the experience over the following months he returned to his formulation again and again to update it with new insights.

Reflection on Exercise 61

You may find this exercise taxing. Your attention may be drawn back to difficult memories and thoughts. This is, of course, perfectly normal. If you find it to be the case for you, each time it happens be mindful of where your attention has gone, and warmly direct it back to the questions you are asking your compassionate mind. If it helps, break off and engage in an exercise such as your soothing rhythm breathing or some form of imagery for a time before returning to the exercise.

Although I would encourage you to do this exercise on your own initially, some people find that it helps later to seek the views of people they trust. How do they see you in light of your influences (past and present) and experiences? If they suggest that you have additional strengths and qualities, make a note of these. Then re-visit the exercise and consider the additional points raised. Let your mind and body absorb these new observations. If you feel comfortable with the statements made about you, add them to the formulation diagram. If you don't feel comfortable writing, for example 'I am kind', it may be helpful to write 'My friend Joe thinks that I am kind'.

Further updates to your formulation

At this point in your journey you may also find it beneficial to engage in Exercise 61 again but this time adding positive influences and experiences you have had and/or currently have. You may wish to note down helpful coping strategies you have discovered and their benefits (as opposed to any drawbacks). All of this updating will hopefully impact on the view you have of yourself and further build your self-confidence.

Finally, as you did previously, you can use this more balanced formulation as a focus for a compassionate letter or further compassionate imagery.

Developing a Template for Self-practice That Will Further Build Your Self-confidence

It is likely that many of the principles and exercises outlined in this book have been helpful to you, though possibly others have been less so. For example, you may have found the 'soothing rhythm breathing' exercise really helpful yet not achieved the same sense of calmness and warmth from engaging with 'place of contentment' imagery. This is absolutely normal and is why the compassionate mind approach introduces a range of different exercises in the hope that you will find some of them of benefit to you.

Throughout this book your attention has been brought to your personal practice summary sheet on page xxviii of the Preface where you were asked to keep a note of how effective you have found the exercises and to record any additional observations you wished to make. Rather than write into the worksheet itself you may have decided to copy the personal practice sheet into your notebook and used this as the place to summarize your experience of exercises.

Have the sheet or notebook to hand as you complete the final exercise of this book in which you will formulate a self-practice system using the exercises that you know work best for you.

Exercise 62: My personal plan for the future

Use worksheet 10 to record the exercises from this book which are most likely to help you continue to build your self-confidence and develop your compassionate mind.

James, whom we first met in Chapter 12, developed a personal practice plan for the future, and this can be used for guidance.

Worksheet 10 : My personal practice plan for the future

Things I have found helpful and would hope to practise daily:

What will help me keep up this practice?

Things that I have found helpful and would hope to practise weekly:

What will help me keep up this practice?

Things that I have found helpful and would hope to practise at certain intervals:

What will help me keep up this practice?

Things that I have found helpful and would hope to practise when times are difficult:

What will help me keep up this practice?

Things that I have found helpful and would hope to practise when things are going well:

What will help me keep up this practice?

Diagram 6: Andy's updated formulation

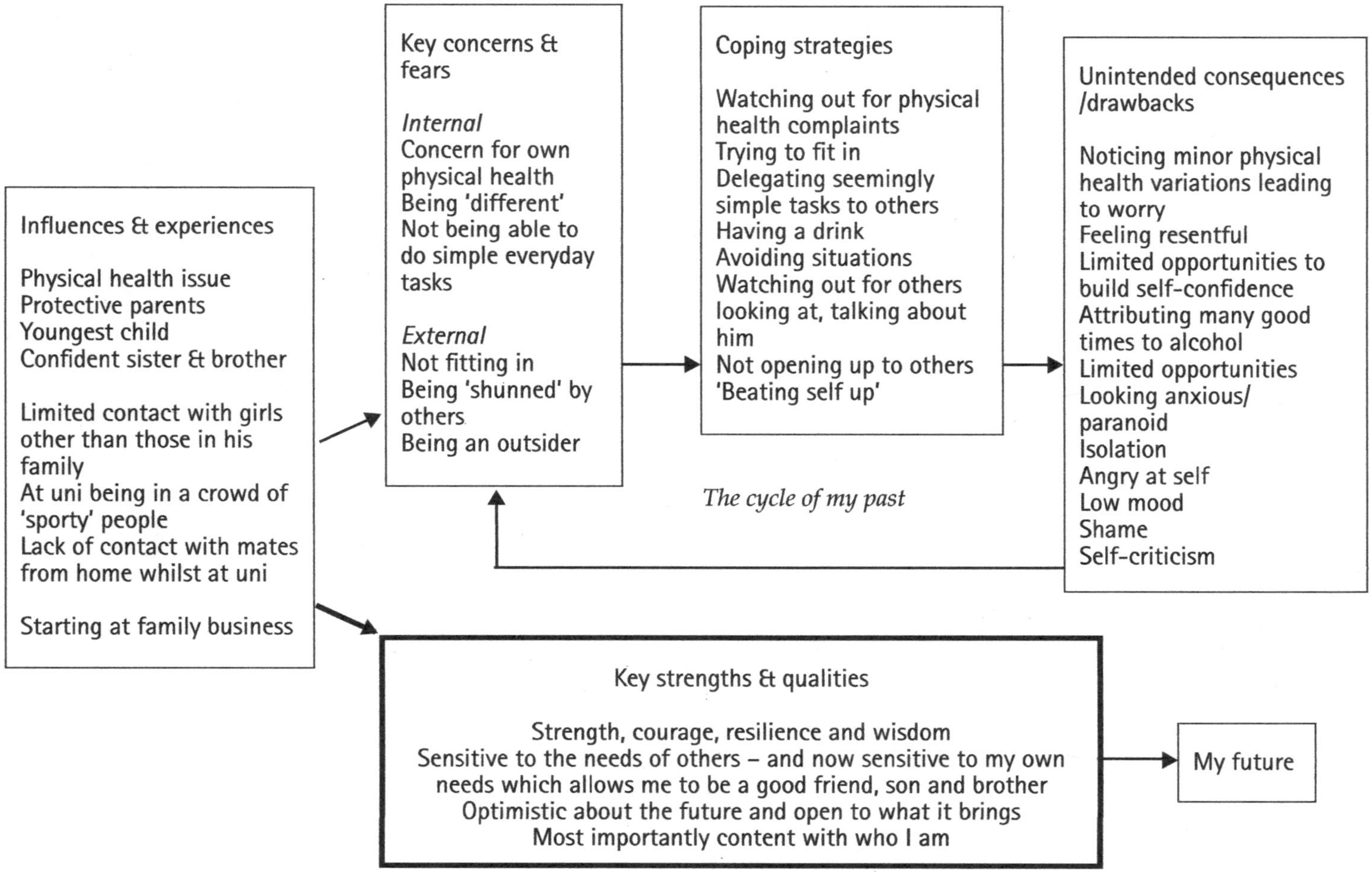

Influences & experiences

Physical health issue
Protective parents
Youngest child
Confident sister & brother

Limited contact with girls other than those in his family
At uni being in a crowd of 'sporty' people
Lack of contact with mates from home whilst at uni

Starting at family business

Key concerns & fears

Internal
Concern for own physical health
Being 'different'
Not being able to do simple everyday tasks

External
Not fitting in
Being 'shunned' by others
Being an outsider

Coping strategies

Watching out for physical health complaints
Trying to fit in
Delegating seemingly simple tasks to others
Having a drink
Avoiding situations
Watching out for others looking at, talking about him
Not opening up to others
'Beating self up'

The cycle of my past

Unintended consequences /drawbacks

Noticing minor physical health variations leading to worry
Feeling resentful
Limited opportunities to build self-confidence
Attributing many good times to alcohol
Limited opportunities
Looking anxious/ paranoid
Isolation
Angry at self
Low mood
Shame
Self-criticism

Key strengths & qualities

Strength, courage, resilience and wisdom
Sensitive to the needs of others – and now sensitive to my own needs which allows me to be a good friend, son and brother
Optimistic about the future and open to what it brings
Most importantly content with who I am

My future

James's personal practice plan for the future

Things I have found helpful and would hope to practise daily:

Mindfulness when I walk the dog – switching my focus from one sense to another.

Towards the end of the walk I will evoke my ideal compassionate self, whose perspective I will take when I look ahead to the rest of the day.

Soothing rhythm breathing just before I go into work.

Asking myself 'What can I do today that will make tomorrow a better day?' after my first hot drink of the day. I will use my compassionate coach imagery to evoke a compassionate mindset before I do this.

What will help me keep up this practice?

Having the prompts of the walk, the drink and going into work will help.

Write this plan up again on a card and keep it in my journal.

Review how I have got along on the first of the month.

Things that I have found helpful and would hope to practise weekly:

On a Sunday I will write a compassionate letter to myself, using imagery first.

On a Saturday morning I will practise my imagery, allowing myself 30 minutes.

In the above exercise I will ask my compassionate coach to help me design a compassionate behavioural experiment, aimed at building my self-confidence, for the week ahead.

What will help me keep up this practice?

I will write it on my calendar till the end of the year.

I will try not to book other things in at those times, and if I do I will move the practice elsewhere and make a note of it.

Things that I have found helpful and would hope to practise at certain intervals:

I will book into my diary one day every two months when I will go for a walk somewhere beautiful and practise mindful walking. When I stop for breaks I will evoke my compassionate coach and, from this perspective, reflect on the time since I last did a weekend walk and look ahead to the weeks before my next one.

At the end of each month I will use chair work to help me see my present situation from both my day-to-day perspective and then from my compassionate coach's perspective – I will set aside evenings on my calendar for this.

What will help me keep up this practice?

Entries on the calendar.

Monthly review points.

Things that I have found helpful and would hope to practise when times are difficult:

All of the above plus:

Compassionate alternative thought worksheets on the days things are difficult.

Review the 'Taking Action' chapter.

Sitting in the presence of my compassionate coach with the difficulties I am having.

If I am having difficulties with someone else, looking at their situation from the ideal compassionate self's perspective – doing this in the evening following any difficulty.

In difficult situations, taking a soothing breath, adjusting my posture and imagining warmth with (if appropriate) a slight smile on my face.

Compassionate letter writing.

Maybe doing slightly different things each day, to help gain a broader and richer compassionate perspective.

What will help me keep up this practice?

Knowing it works.

Reading my letters to myself to reinforce this.

Things that I have found helpful and would hope to practise when things are going well:

Savour the experience.

If someone has said something positive or acted towards me positively, making a note of it on my formulation.

Updating my formulation at set intervals.

What will help me keep up this practice?

Slowing down and noticing positive experiences.

Keeping my journal with me as a reminder.

Doing all of the above will help me further tune my mind to increased self-confidence.

Reflection on Exercise 62

Remember that this is a compassionate plan to help further build both your self-confidence and your compassionate mind. You can adjust and amend it, in light of new experiences, at any time.

Also remember that you are planning here for what you *hope* to do. Life gets in the way for all of us sometimes. We can get caught up in all manner of things that divert us from our original aim. This is often most true in the early days, years and months of self-practice. When you do notice that you have wandered away from your plan, re-familiarize yourself with the work you have done to date. Then reflect on why you may have veered away from your plan, as this may give you some insight into the obstacles that have been raised and help you focus your mind on how to negotiate them. Finally, rethink your plan. If necessary, adjust it and then resume your journey.

Final Thoughts

As mentioned at the start of this book, in years gone by I would have been unable to hand over the final draft of this book without experiencing crippling self-criticism. As a young adult I was convinced that if people truly knew me they wouldn't like me – or at best would be indifferent. My mind was plagued by self-doubt, regrets, worries, and at times I was emotionally all over the place.

It's not that I think I am brilliant now – it's something better than that. I can warmly accept myself, warts and all. I can be compassionate towards myself and also feel more 'connected' with others. This sense that 'we are all in it together' is very different from the treadmill of constantly comparing myself, favourably or (more commonly) not, to other people. This has made me more self-confident and ultimately more content.

I wouldn't claim that *all* of this has been down to the application of the compassionate mind approach to my life. I had travelled some way down the path to self-confidence and self-compassion already, but this approach certainly accelerated the process. My continued practice helps me maintain a healthy state of mind by being more resilient to life's knocks.

It takes time to forge a new path. We have to overcome obstacles, negotiate a tendency to walk the more familiar route, be courageous. Having said that, I think – and most importantly *know* from my own experience – that the rewards are worth it.

I sincerely wish you all the best in the next stage of your journey.

References

Chapter 1

A seminal book on compassion, covering why and how to develop it for ourselves: P. Gilbert, *The Compassionate Mind* (Constable and Robinson, 2009).

Chapter 2

On the threat system: R. F. Baumeister, E. Bratslavsky, C. Finkenauer and K. D. Vohs, 'Bad is Stronger than Good', *Review of General Psychology*, 5, 2001, 323–70.

On how our old brain and new brain can conflict: N. F. Dixon, *Our Own Worst Enemy* (Routledge, 1987).

On the science behind the three emotion regulation systems: R. A. Depue and J. V. Morrone-Strupinsky, 'A Neurobehavioural Model of Affiliative Bonding', *Behavioral and Brain Sciences*, 28, 2005, 313–95.

On the importance of good attachment with our care-givers: S. Gerhardt, *Why Love Matters: How Affection Shapes a Baby's Brain* (Bruner-Routledge, 2004).

On modern society and how it intentionally over-stimulates the drive and acquisition system: J. M. Twenge, B. Gentile, C. N. DeWall, D. S. Ma, K. Lacefield and D. R. Schurtz, 'Birth cohort increases in psychopathology amongst young Americans 1938–2007: A cross-temporal meta-analysis of the MMPI', *Clinical Psychology Review*, 30, 2010, 145–154.

Chapter 3

On shame: P. Gilbert, 'The Evolution of Shame as a Marker of Relationship

Security', in J. L. Tracy, R. W. Robins and J. P. Tangney (eds), *The Self-conscious Emotions: Theory and Research* (Guilford Press, 2007), 283–309.

On reflected shame: J. Sanghera, *Shame* (Hodder & Stoughton, 2007).

On self-criticism: P. Gilbert and C. Irons, 'Focused Therapies and Compassionate Mind Training for Shame and Self-attacking', in P. Gilbert (ed.), *Compassion: Conceptualisations, Research and Use in Psychotherapy* (Routledge, 2005), 263–325.

P. Gilbert, M. W. Baldwin, C. Irons, J. R. Baccus and M. Palmer, 'Self-criticism and Self-warmth: An Imagery Study Exploring their Relation to Depression', *Journal of Cognitive Psychotherapy*, 20 (2), 2006, 183–200.

On the different forms of perfectionism: D. M. Dunkley, K. R. Blankstein, D. C. Zuroff, S. Lecce and D. Hui, 'Self-critical and Personal Standards: Factors of Perfectionism Located within the Five-factor Model of Personality', *Personality and Individual Differences*, 40, 2006, 409–20.

On motivations behind the goals we set: B. M. Dykman, 'Integrating Cognitive and Motivational Factors in Depression: Initial Tests of a Goal-orientation Approach', *Journal of Personality and Social Psychology*, 74 (1), 1998, 139–58.

On the importance of self-compassion: K. D. Neff, *Self-Compassion: Stop Beating Yourself Up and Leave Insecurity Behind* (HarperCollins, 2011).

Chapter 5

Views of compassion: R. Davidson and A. Harrington (eds), *Visions of Compassion: Western Scientists and Tibetan Buddhists Examine Human Nature* (Oxford University Press, 2002).

On social mentalities: P. Gilbert, *Psychotherapy and Counselling for Depression* (Sage, 2007, 3rd edn); P. Gilbert, 'Social Mentalities: Internal

'Social' Conflicts and the Role of Inner Warmth and Compassion in Cognitive Therapy', in P. Gilbert and K. G. Bailey (eds), *Genes on the Couch: Explorations in Evolutionary Psychotherapy* (Brenner-Routledge, 2005), 118–50.

On attachment and brain development: L. Cozolino, *The Neuroscience of Human Relationships: Attachment and the Developing Brain* (Norton, 2007).

Chapter 6

On the experience of stress in response to compassion: H. Rockliff, P. Gilbert, K. McEwan, S. Lightman and D. Glover, 'An Exploration of Heart-rate Variability and Salivary Cortisol Responses to Compassion-focused Imagery', *Journal of Clinical Neuropsychiatry*, 5, 2008, 132–39.

Chapter 7

On mindfulness: J. Kabat-Zinn, *Coming to Our Senses: Healing Ourselves and the World through Mindfulness* (Piatkus, 2005); J. Kabat-Zinn, *Mindfulness for Beginners* (Sounds True, 2006).

On mindfulness and self-compassion: C. K. Germer, *The Mindful Path to Self-compassion* (Guilford Press, 2009).

Chapter 9

On compassionate mind training: P. Gilbert and C. Irons, 'Focused Therapies and Compassionate Mind Training for Shame and Self-attacking', in P. Gilbert (ed.), *Compassion: Conceptualisations, Research and Use in Psychotherapy* (Routledge, 2005), 263–325.

On Compassion Focused Therapy (CFT): P. Gilbert, *Compassion-focused Therapy: Distinctive Features* (Routledge, 2010).

On 'perfect nurturer' imagery: D. A. Lee, 'The Perfect Nurturer: A Model to Develop a Compassionate Mind Within the Context of Cognitive

Therapy', in P. Gilbert (ed.), *Compassion: Conceptualisations, Research and Use in Psychotherapy* (Routledge, 2005), 326–51.

Chapter 10

On our tendency to think in certain ways: C. Fine, *A Mind of Its Own: How your Brain Distorts and Deceives* (Icon Books, 2007).

Chapter 11

On the use of writing as a means of promoting well-being: J. W. Pennebaker, *Writing to Heal: A Guided Journal for Recovering from Trauma and Emotional Upheaval* (New Harbinger, 2004).

On random acts of kindness: S. Hynbomirsky, R. M. Sheldon and D. Schlade 'Pursuing Happiness: The Architecture of Sustainable Change', in *Review of General Psychology*, 9, 205, 113–31.

Chapter 13

On assertiveness: D. Johnson, *Reaching Out: Interpersonal Effectiveness and Self-actualization* (Allyn & Bacon, 2008, 10th edn).

On acceptance: S. Hayes and S. Smith, *Get Out of Your Mind and Into Your Life* (New Harbinger, 2005); T. Brach, *Radical Acceptance: Embracing Your Life with the Heart of a Buddha* (Bantam, 2004).

Useful Resources

Further Reading

You will find listed below a number of publications that may be of interest to you. Some of them are referred to within this book while others I would recommend as further reading should you wish to explore a particular topic in depth.

Acceptance and Commitment Therapy (ACT): Steven Hayes and Spencer Smith, *Get Out of Your Mind and Into Your Life* (New Harbinger, 2005).

Anger: Russell Kolts, *The Compassionate Mind Approach to Managing Your Anger* (Robinson, 2012).

Anxiety and social confidence: Lynne Henderson, *Improving Social Confidence and Reducing Shyness Using Compassion Focused Therapy* (Robinson, 2010);
Susan Jeffers, *Feel the Fear and Do It Anyway* (Random House, 1987).

Compassion: Christopher K. Germer, *The Mindful Path to Self-compassion* (Guilford Press, 2009); Paul Gilbert, *Compassion: Conceptualisations, Research and Use in Psychotherapy* (Routledge, 2005), and *The Compassionate Mind* (Constable and Robinson, 2009).

Self-Compassion: Kristin Neff, *Self Compassion: Stop Beating Yourself Up and Leave Insecurity Behind* (HarperCollins, 2011).

Depression: Paul Gilbert, *Overcoming Depression: A Self-help Guide to Using Cognitive Behavioural Techniques* (Robinson, 2009, 3rd edn).

Difficulties associated with eating: Susan Albers, *Eating Mindfully: How to End Mindless Eating and Enjoy a Balanced Relationship With Food* (New Harbinger, 2003);

Kenneth Goss, *The Compassionate Mind Approach to Beating Overeating* (Constable and Robinson, 2010).

General self-help: Elizabeth Lesser, *Broken Open: How Difficult Times Can Help Us Grow* (Villard Books, 2004).

Science of the brain: John Arden and Lloyd Linford, *Brain-based Therapy with Adults* (Wiley, 2009); John Arden, *Rewire Your Brain* (Wiley, 2010); Susan Begley, *The Plastic Mind* (Constable, 2009).

Shame: Paul Gilbert and Bernice Andrews, *Shame: Interpersonal Behaviour, Psychopathology, and Culture* (Oxford University Press, 1998); Jasvinder Sanghera, *Shame* (Hodder & Stoughton, 2007).

Trauma Deborah Lee with Sophie James, *The Compassionate Mind Approach to Recovering from Trauma* (Robinson, 2012).

Organizations and Websites

The following organizations and websites may be of help and/or interest to you:

British Association for Behavioural & Cognitive Psychotherapies (www.babcp.com)
Predominantly set up for therapists, the website includes a section for the public which contains information on Cognitive Behaviour Therapy (CBT), self-help and how to find a private therapist.

Centre for Compassion and Altruism Research (http://ccare.stanford.edu/)
Set up by Professor James Doty for international work for the advancement of compassion.

Compassionate Mind Foundation (www.compassionatemind.co.uk)
In 2007, Paul Gilbert and a number of colleagues (including myself) set up a charity called the Compassionate Mind Foundation. On this website,

you will find various learning resources and details of other sites which look at different aspects of compassion. You will also find a lot of material that you can use for meditation on compassion.

Living Life to the Full (www.livinglifetothefull.com)
Set up by Dr Chris Williams and based on the principles of Cognitive Behaviour Therapy, this website provides access to practical and user-friendly training in life skills. Web-based sessions focus on such areas as mood, anxiety, sleep and confidence.

Mind (www.mind.org.uk; tel. 0300 123 3393)
Mind is a charity aimed at promoting 'better mental health'. It provides high-quality information and advice on a wide range of mental-health issues.

Mind & Life Institute (www.mindandlife.org)
The Dalai Lama has forged relationships with Western scientists to research and develop a more compassionate way of living. More information can be found on the website.

MoodGYM (www.moodgym.anu.edu.au)
Based on the principles of Cognitive Behaviour Therapy(CBT), MoodGYM was designed at the Centre for Mental Health Research of the Australian National University and is a free web program designed to help prevent depression.

The Samaritans (www.samaritans.org.uk; tel. 08457 90 90 90)
The Samaritans offer 24-hour support over the telephone for anybody in distress.

Self-Compassion (www.self-compassion.org)
Dr Kristin Neff is one of the leading researchers into self-compassion.

There are many more websites you can explore if you go to the website section of the Compassionate Mind Foundation site.

Index